SOAP MAKING RECIPES

The Complete Beginner's Guide to Natural Soap Making

(Your Complete Step-by-step Guide to Make Organic Soaps at Home)

Jesus Cutter

Published by Oliver Leish

Jesus Cutter

All Rights Reserved

Soap Making Recipes: The Complete Beginner's Guide to Natural Soap Making (Your Complete Step-by-step Guide to Make Organic Soaps at Home)

ISBN 978-1-77485-089-3

All rights reserved. No part of this guide may be reproduced in any form without permission in writing from the publisher except in the case of brief quotations embodied in critical articles or reviews.

Legal & Disclaimer

The information contained in this book is not designed to replace or take the place of any form of medicine or professional medical advice. The information in this book has been provided for educational and entertainment purposes only.

The information contained in this book has been compiled from sources deemed reliable, and it is accurate to the best of the Author's knowledge; however, the Author cannot guarantee its accuracy and validity and cannot be held liable for any errors or omissions. Changes are periodically made to this book. You must consult your doctor or get professional medical advice before using any of the suggested remedies, techniques, or information in this book.

Upon using the information contained in this book, you agree to hold harmless the Author from and against any damages, costs, and expenses, including any legal fees potentially resulting from the application of any of the information provided by this guide. This disclaimer applies to any damages or injury caused by the use and application, whether directly or indirectly, of any advice or information presented, whether for breach of contract, tort, negligence, personal injury, criminal intent, or under any other cause of action.

You agree to accept all risks of using the information presented inside this book. You need to consult a professional medical practitioner in order to ensure you are both able and healthy enough to participate in this program.

Table of Contents

INTRODUCTION 1

CHAPTER 1: HOW PROFITABLE IS THE SOAP MAKING BUSINESS? 4

CHAPTER 2: GETTING STARTED 11

CHAPTER 3: EVERY SOAP MAKER SHOULD HAVE THIS 20

CHAPTER 4: SOAP MAKING EQUIPMENT 40

CHAPTER 5: SOAP MAKING - THE BASICS 47

CHAPTER 6: WHAT KIND OF "SOAPIE" ARE YOU? 58

CHAPTER 7: HISTORY OF SOAP 63

CHAPTER 8: HAND SANITIZER 84

CHAPTER 9: HOW TO KEEP CUSTOMERS COMING BACK .. 99

CHAPTER 10: SOAP MAKING TOOLS 112

CHAPTER 11: BEST HOMEMADE SOAP RECIPES 135

CHAPTER 12: SAPONIFICATION GUIDE 147

CHAPTER 13: TIME FOR SOME HOMEMADE RECIPES! ... 152

1.) Tea Tree and Activated Charcoal Soap – 152
Pure Coconut Oil Soap – 156

2.) Aloe Vera Soap 160

3.) Coffee Soap – 163

5.) HONEY OATMEAL SOAP – 165

6.) Lemon Green Tea Soap – 169

Coconut Milk Shampoo Bars- 171

7.) Dandelions Soap Bar – 174

8.) Honey and Milk Soap – 177

9.) Creamy Avocado Soap Bar – 180

10.) Lavender Lotion Bar – 183

11.) Orange Clove Soap Bar – 185

Vanilla and Brown Sugar Soap – 187

12.) Banana and Yogurt Soap Bar – 189

CHAPTER 14: RECIPES 194

CONCLUSION 201

Introduction

The Babylons made soap during 2000 BC. It was formed from ashes and fats from the food they ate. During the Roman era, soap was made from Goat and Wood Ash. Throughout history, each era brought its own different soap making methods.

Sodium based alkali is now the method we use today for true soap making.

Once it caught on, it was no longer a novel idea to use for cleaning. It became a necessity. The industry began in Italy and France. It later spread throughout Europe after the French discovered the use of olive oil instead of animal fat.

A Swedish chemist, Carl Wilhelm Scheele, discovered how to make and extract the glycerine from the soap by cooking it. Glycerine is extracted and used in countless products today. In fact it is considered to be more valuable than the soap itself.

As people began to take cleanliness more seriously and realized that it was a successful way to control disease, more and more companies began massive campaigns to advertise their soap.

Companies' such as Pears and Lever began in the industry and are still around today.

Soap making has changed a lot since this time, yet the methods for creating true soap has not. With all of the alternatives to natural soap, we now spend much more time choosing the right soap for our skin and ethical views. This is getting more difficult with all of the chemical substitutes for real soap on the market.

The easiest and most cost effective way to find soap that suits your skin and values, are to discover soap making for yourself. You choose your oils, your scent and the color you prefer. Soap making is fun and easy when you have guidance and learn from an experienced teacher.

Chapter 1: How Profitable Is The Soap Making Business?

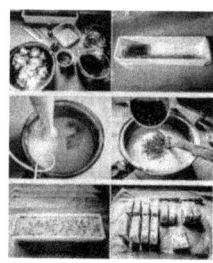

The soap business is profitable, you can make money selling soap, well there's the big 'BUT,' you have to get out of the mindset of a hobby if it's your hobby. And you want to make a few bucks extra from it, then that is perfect as long as you have acknowledged this before you start.

For any profit you want to make from the business, you must first treat it as a business. You have to get to the point where you're efficient at it; you can do it quickly and repeat the process over and over again; for your profit come to in, what you produce need to be repeated. So make every process, every part of your process repeatable. And that will help.

The more efficient you get at something, the more money you're going to make on it. The higher you buy in bulk (bulk oils, bulk fragrances, bulk essential oils) and all that, the more you make, the cheaper each product gets for you, which gives you a higher markup of more profit. The first rule in business is making a profit, not just covering costs or losing money.

Benefits and Drawbacks of Starting Soap Business from Home

First, everybody wants to know the monetary and economic side of things. So, number one, you will be losing a lot of money, and that's because the soap gear and oils, the fragrance oils, the cutter, are not cheap, they're very expensive. If you want to start making cold process, it's going to be pretty expensive for you, and that's because you will buy things like the soap molds, the silicone mold for you to mold if it's a wooden one. You're going to need packaging, color variants, sodium hydroxide, also known as lye, and they are pretty expensive. There are a few things that you can get locally that might be less expensive because of the shipping.

The second thing that has to do with money is that you should start with at least $1,000 for materials, or $2,000. If you want to make this a business and you want to save money from your materials, always buy in bulk; most of these tips come from people who are making thousands of dollars a month with selling their soaps. Even though you don't imagine yourself making that much soap, like a 50 pounds coconut oil barrel might seem too much for you, but once you start making soap, you'll keep on making, so it's going to be a lot less expensive than buying in smaller quantities.

The third thing I want to tell you about is, you will spend a lot of time marketing, like 80% of a soap business is marketing, 20% is for soap making because right now, there are lots of soap makers. However, there are not enough soap makers for the entire world. There is still quite a lot of variety for you to choose from. In this type of business, you need to make yourself known because it's something that people put on their skins.

Soap Making Equipment Needed To Start

1. The first thing you're going to need is a scale; it's very important because you have to weigh your ingredients very precisely to your liking if you want your bars to come out perfect.

2. The thermometer, you have to have a good scale and a good thermometer if you want quality soap bars. These two are essential.

3. Next, we're going to talk about the mixing utensils; make sure it's stainless steel; you can get a variety of spoons. Preferably the ladle when you have to mix it into a plastic bowl to add coloring. So that's when you use the ladle. You can use just a regular spoon to mix it to bring it to trace, or you can buy a little mixer, make sure you get one with stainless steel blades. When you have little individual molds, it's easier if you can spoon it into the mold, and some molds have even a different shape; it just helps you be a little neat and tidy.

4. Next, we're going to talk about bowls. If you are making soap in large quantities, you are going to be needing a big shallow bowl. Again, it has to be stainless steel or plastic.

5. Also, you're going to need some little tubs, you know these are cottage cheese tubs just get as many as you want,

especially if you want to make colored soap.

6. Furthermore, we're going to talk about the lye. You can use it to make bagels, and after that is the variety of essential oils. You can use whatever fragrance you enjoy. The fragrance bottles are 0.3 ounces or 10 milliliters, that's the amount you put in your soap recipe, whichever recipe you're following. This makes the soap mildly fragrant. It'll be just right.

7. Next is the soap molds that you pour the soap into, preferably the sillcone molds. They are very easy to pop the bars out when it's time; you can make cute little shapes, which makes it so much fun to make your soap. Again, choose the shapes you like, or, if you want the standard bar soaps, which is old fashioned, they're very flexible, nice things that last. They are durable; you can wash them. They're easy to store; you don't have to

worry about them; just pile them up and put them somewhere.

8. The needlepoint plastic that you can see through it is also required. It's airy. So you need to put it into your cardboard box to be able to lay your bars on it,

9. Towels are also essential in your soap making journey, just use the regular household towels, dish towels, and wash them when you are done.

Chapter 2: Getting Started

In order to understand soap making to a level where you can easily create your own soaps, you need to first understand the terminology that is used in the process. The terminology is the same around the world, so by mastering this part of the soap-making process, you will easily be able to look for any further questions that you may have and to connect with other soap-making lovers.

Trace

You will come across this term throughout your entire soap-making process. When you make soap, you are combining oils (of your choice) and lye water, in order to get the right consistency for the soap that you are trying to make. Trace refers to the quality to which you have mixed the oil and the water together; you can either have a thin trace or a thick trace.

When making soap, you will usually use a hand mixer (hand-held blender) to combine the two together. It makes the process quick and easy and is a great tool to ensure that everything is properly blended together.

Trace refers to whether or not you can write your name with the blender when you pull it out of the soap mixture. You can think of this as similar to when you are trying to make whipped cream to its proper consistency. If you can trace your name, this is a thick trace. If you cannot, then it is a thin trace.

In general, you want to ensure that you have a thick trace so that the soap looks smooth and beautiful when you are done making it. If you were to pour the mixture with the oil and the water divided, your soap would not have the right consistency, which means that it would split as it dries. However, as you become more professional in your soap making, you will be able to play around with trace to create beautiful soap designs.

Gel Phase

This is a special consistency of soap that reaches a temperature of 180 degrees Fahrenheit. In this state, the soap consistency is reminiscent of a gel, meaning that much of it will have a clear texture. If you wish to make this kind of soap, it will have a very bright appearance and will also be much brighter in color. On the contrary, the usual consistency of soap is creamy in texture, with less of a color impact. Which one you use depends on what kind of style you are looking to have in the end.

This phase is not obligatory when you are making soap; you can simply go for the standard creamy texture if you prefer.

However, gel soap is easier to demold and to cut, which is also another benefit that soap makers look for. There is also no difference in quality between the two types of soap. As long as the ingredients themselves are of the highest quality possible, then the end product will be of high quality as well.

Curing

When you are done making soap, it is usually ready to use after a few days in the mold. However, if you want to create more structured soap with a firmer texture, then it is a good idea to leave the soap to cure for about three weeks. During this time, the excess water will evaporate from the soap, making it harder and also more durable for use. Soap that is much harder in texture will release its oils in smaller quantities, making it last longer; something that your customers will certainly appreciate.

Calculating Lye

A lye calculator is a tool that is used when making soap through the cold process (without heating the ingredients). This device helps you to calculate the amount of oil that is currently in your soap mixture. You can even enter your desired number and then use the lye calculator to work on the ingredients until you reach your desired amount. It will take you a few tries before you are able to use the lye calculator properly, but it is one of the most important tools for soap makers.

Soda Ash

Soda ash occurs when you make a mistake in the production of your soap. Although it will not ruin the soap in terms of its use and efficiency, it does ruin it visually. If the lye is not properly balanced within your soap, then carbon dioxide from the outside will enter parts of your soap, causing them to become white and foggy.

There is no way to fix this once the soap is dry, but you can still use the soap if you wish to. Also, the soap bars will likely crumble once you start using them and when they come into contact with water. As a result, you will not experience the soft creaminess of a well-created soap bar.

Safety When Working with Lye

Lye is one of the key ingredients for anyone who may be working with soap. However, in order to be safe around lye, you need to understand how to use it and what kind of equipment you will need to keep on hand as you work.

The reason why is because it is extremely corrosive. It is very dangerous both for your skin and for your eyes, and should of course never be swallowed or deeply breathed in. To start ensuring that you are truly safe around lye, make sure that family members are at a distance, and that there are no children or pets nearby. If there does happen to be someone else working with you on the production of soap, make sure that they are also wearing all of the necessary protective equipment.

Gloves

High-quality gloves are essential when you are working with the liquids that go inside soap. Make sure that you get the proper laboratory gloves that go all the way up to your elbows. They need to be able to cover a large surface of your skin, so that you can stay protected in case any splashes occur while you work.

Goggles

Another piece of very important equipment are of course goggles. Since we mentioned that lye is very dangerous for your eyes, you need to protect them with the help of professional goggles. Once again, choose the ones that would be used in laboratories, because they are the most likely to have the high standard of quality that can truly protect your eyes.

Protective Clothing

As you work on developing your own style of soap, there will almost certainly be splashes and mistakes along the way, and you really need to make sure that you prepare for them so that you don't suffer any injuries. In order to do this, you need to make sure that the clothing you are wearing is the kind that will be able to protect you against accidental burns. Choose clothes that have thick textures, with long sleeves and long pants. Also, make sure that you are not wearing slippers, but instead ensure that you are wearing proper shoes that will also protect your toes.

Face Mask

A good face mask will protect you from any fumes that may be coming up from your soap mixture. This is especially important if you have any kind of allergies or perhaps asthma. You need to ensure that you protect your lungs from any substances that might cause them harm. This is especially true if you intend to be working on soap for a long period of time, because small injuries here and there could eventually pile up into a serious problem.

Chapter 3: Every Soap Maker Should Have This

Equipment used in making soap

So you were so propelled by the primary section that you need to run directly out and buy the entirety of the materials you need right? Indeed, this part and the following will assist you with making your shopping list and furthermore let you know where you might need to go to get the things you need. Contrasted with numerous different artworks, you needn't bother with much hardware to cause soap and quite a bit of what you to do require is reasonable. Indeed, you may as of now have quite a bit of what you need in your kitchen.

Significant security note-it is pivotal that once you utilize an instrument for soap causing you to don't utilize it for cooking or some other action. A portion of the synthetic compounds utilized in soap causing are noxious whenever ingested and can to consume the skin. Ensure you store your soap making utensils independently from your kitchen-use utensils.

While picking your apparatuses it is essential to pick hardware that isn't made of aluminum, metal, or bronze when making soap. These metals respond contrarily to lye and will present wellbeing risks and won't produce generally excellent final products for your soap. Tempered steel, glass, and polish are acceptable decisions.

First here is a rundown of the fundamentals that don't need a lot of clarification:

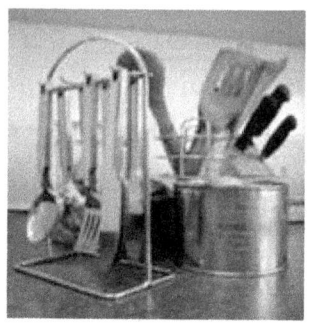

☐Freezer paper or saran wrap (not wax paper) to cover your work surface and line the form if necessary

☐6-8 inch steel blade for cutting soap on the off chance that you are not utilizing a form

☐Drying rack to permit your soap to fix

☐Droppers or pipettes to include shading and scent

☐Rubber spatula to mix

☐Stainless steel spoons to mix

☐Stainless steel race to blend

☐ Bowls

☐ 4-cup glass measure to guarantee you are including the perfect measure of every fixing

☐ Waterproof advanced thermometer ideally produced using treated steel and at any rate 5 inches in length

☐ Rubbing liquor in a splash bottle

☐ Crockpot (discretionary)

☐ Double evaporator (discretionary)

☐ Microwave (discretionary)

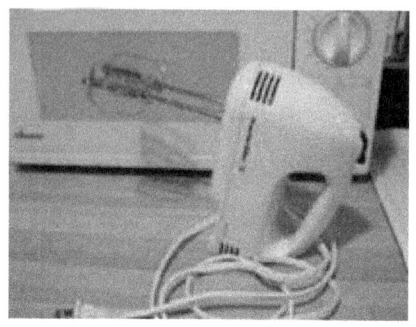

There are a couple different bits of gear you will require which require a smidgen more conversation with the goal for you to have the option to settle on an informed decision at the store. The first of these things is a blender. You may conclude that hand blending works for you, especially in the event that you need to consolidate soap making with your everyday exercise. In any case, for some, blending soap for near an hour with the goal for it to completely begin the saponification cycle won't prompt individual satisfaction. On the off chance that you are one of those individuals, you have several choices to consider. An electric hand blender can be utilized yet has its disadvantages. Utilizing this strategy there is an inclination for a ton of air to get included into the blend. This can cause some huge issues with the group of soap including have air pockets all through the completed item. The utilization of a stick or inundation blender is energetically suggested. Search for one that has a basic plan with cutting edges that interface with the blender and a strong part behind the edges. You need to search for a low, short end on your blender (around the sharp edge zone). Additionally, discover a blender that has a smooth base edge. Abstain from picking one with scores or edges. Try not to stress over having a few speed settings; it won't make any difference as you will beat it or utilizing it in the off position. By utilizing a stick blender you can chop down the time it takes to arrive at a follow essentially. We are talking from 45 minutes down to 5. Critical. Some soap plans tend to isolate and the danger of this event is significantly less when utilizing a stick blender. So now that the delights of the stick blender have been shared, there is an admonition. You might need to mix by hand or utilize a normal electric hand blender when making your first couple of clumps. This will permit you to obviously observe the stages your soap is experiencing and, specifically, recognize when you have arrived at the follow stage. It is extremely simple to get a bogus follow when utilizing a stick blender

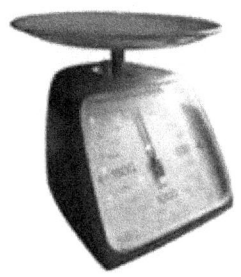

Another significant bit of gear is a scale. When estimating elements for a soap formula the estimations, especially lye and water, must be careful. More careful than

estimating cups would be without a doubt. Estimating with a scale will make it more probable that the soap making cycle will be without glitch. It is additionally more secure as the synthetic substances utilized will respond in the anticipated manner that you have made arrangements for. At the point when you are buying a scale you need to search for a few things. Initially, you need it to be computerized so you get extremely accurate readings. It will likewise be helpful on the off chance that it can disclose to you loads in Metric and English estimations. This will spare the way toward changing over estimations from plans written in metric units into English terms and the other way around. Size is another thought. You need your scale to have a useable surface of in any event six inches square. The scale's unit of graduation is vital. Soap making requires estimating some exceptionally modest quantities so search for a scale that measures in 1 gram and .1 ounce increases.

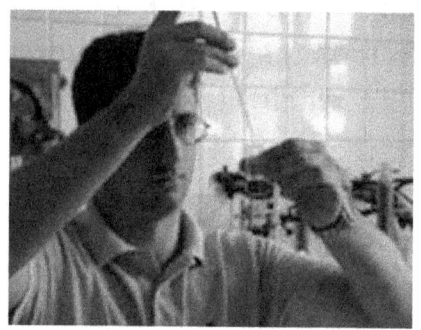

Since we are working with acids and bases that can be hurtful when they come in contact on the skin if not killed, it is helpful to test the pH of your soap sooner or later. On a pH scale, numbers under 7 connote acids and numbers over 7 mean a soluble base. It is alluring for soap to have a pH of somewhere in the range of 7 and 10. Except if you purchase truly costly lab-quality pH testing hardware, you are left with two or three choices to test pH, none of which give us a very precise perusing however some data is superior to no data. The first, and most conventional test, is to put a drop of soap on your tongue. On the off chance that it destroys like an electric stun, you realize that the lye has not been killed and you have to continue blending or cooking so as to cut the pH down and make the soap safe. The "hand test" can likewise be utilized. At the point when the soap is done, wash your hands with it. In the event that it gives little foam and causes skin disturbance, the pH is likely not inside the sheltered range. In the event that these thoughts are not engaging you, go on an outing to the drug store where you can buy pH strips. To utilize these, place a drop of water on your soap and afterward put the test strip on the water. Since this tests the pH of the water and not the cemented (or semi-set) soap, it isn't totally exact however you do show signs of improvement thought of where the soap is at. Another apparatus that can be utilized is phenolphthalein. This is a fluid that you drop in limited quantities onto the soap. On the off chance that the fluid is clear or light pink you are good to go. In the event that it is a more obscure shading, you have to proceed with the saponification cycle to make it safe. Phenolphthalein is most effectively found at a store that sells pool supplies as it is additionally used to test the wellbeing of swimming water.

Soap molds are likely the best time and intriguing bits of hardware you will look for. Soap molds come in all shapes and sizes. Some are modest and some are out and out expensive. There are a couple general courses you can take to pick a form. You could choose to buy singular molds to empty the soap straightforwardly into. Despite the fact that those work very well for the liquefy and pour strategy, it doesn't turn out to be very also with the virus cycle as they are more hard to protect. You could likewise buy a wooden shape called a soap portion or line a portion skillet with cling wrap and utilize that (recollect not to utilize it for cooking after). When the soap as solidified, the soap can be taken out from the shape and cut. There are an assortment of hardware choices for soap cutting. These include:

☐ Smooth edge cutters

☐ Krinkle edge shaper

☐ Single bar cutting box

☐ Soap edger

It likewise simple to make your own soap cutting box utilizing a miter box. Here is how:

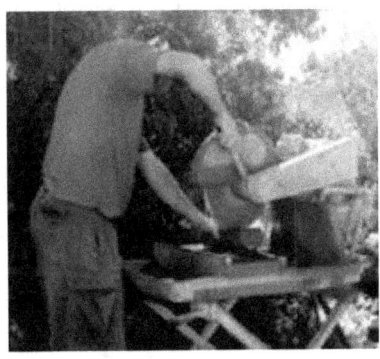

1. Gather materials

☐ Handsaw

☐ Ten 1-inch screws

☐ Screwdriver

☐ ½ inch by 4-inch poplar wood strips. Purchase enough length so you have the length of your miter box times two in addition to eight inches

☐ 1x2 inch wood strips. Purchase enough so you have the length of your miter box times two in addition to eight inches.

☐ Wooden miter box

☐ Electric drill

2. Cut two lengths of the poplar wood to a similar length as the miter box.

3. Cut two lengths of the 1x2 woods strips to a similar length as the miter box.

4. Drill three uniformly separated pilot openings through the 1x2 strips.

5. Drill gaps in similar places somewhat through the poplar strips.

6. Screw the 1x2 and poplar strips together

7. Place the two side strips in the miter box

8. Measure the opening between the different sides. This must be definite as your end pieces need fit snuggly. This keeps soap from spilling out of the shape.

9. cut the poplar and 1x2 strips to the estimation made in the last stride

10. Drill pilot gaps and append the 1x2 wood strips to the poplar strips utilizing screws.

11. Put the pieces into the miter box.

12. Notice that you can change the size of your form by moving the end sorts further separated or closer out.

Your last form choice is to get inventive and go insane. Here are some out of the container thoughts:

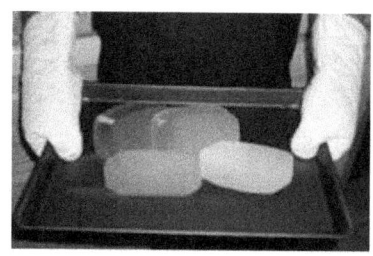

☐ PVC pipe

☐ Pringles can

☐ Cocoa can

☐ Silicone cake molds

☐ Candy molds

☐ Tupperware

- [ ] Shallow dish (you can remove singular shapes with dough shapers)
- [ ] Mini portion container
- [ ] Tin can
- [ ] Box
- [ ] Yogurt compartments
- [ ] Fluted frozen yogurt dishes
- [ ] Muffin container
- [ ] Margarine compartments
- [ ] Mail tubes
- [ ] Toilet paper rolls
- [ ] Paper towel rolls

If all else fails about whether an item can be utilized as a soap shape or not, check the compartment to check whether it is dishwasher as well as microwave safe. In the event that it is, this is a decent pointer than it tends to be utilized. Remember additionally that a shape with one end bigger than the other will deliver the soap all the more effectively after it is solidified.

If you are utilizing a non-customary compartment, it tends to be trying to make sense of exactly how much soap to make to fill it. Fortunately, there is a generally simple approach to discover this data.

Begin by filling a form with water and unloading the water into a fluid measure.

Measure the measure of water in ounces that the compartment held and duplicate that by 1.8 (the quantity of cubic crawls in an ounce of water).

Multiply this number by .40 to decide how much soap oil you should place in the formula to fill the compartment.

Multiply that by the number of compartments you have.

Multiply the measure of soap oils in ounces into the rates of oil in your formula. For instance, if you need 38 ounces of soap oils and your formula calls for 35% olive oil, you will utilize 13.3 ounces of olive oil in your formula (38 x .35).

Since you will utilize synthetic concoctions, lye specifically, the utilization of wellbeing gear is critical to forestall genuine injury. The accompanying wellbeing devices are enthusiastically suggested:

☐ Safety goggles when utilizing lye

☐ Rubber gloves when utilizing lye

☐ Apron

☐ Vinegar and milk to kill lye spills

☐ Table covering, ideally one that can be discarded after each utilization (paper, plastic garbage sack, dollar store decorative liner)

A large portion of the materials referenced in this section can be found by setting off to your neighborhood market, tool shop, cooking store, or enormous box store. If you need to get extravagant with your molds, an excursion to an art store, for example, Ben Franklin's, A.C. Moore, or Michaels would get you what you need. On the off chance that you need to spare yourself from the problem of heading to a few spots, you can buy what you need effectively from the Internet. Most sites won't just sell hardware yet will likewise sell spices, oils, flavors, aromas, and bundling. On the off chance that you are hoping to make a lot of soaps, there are sites where you can buy hardware and fixings in mass permitting you to spare a lot of cash. Here is a short rundown of certain sites where soap causing supplies to can be acquired at sensible costs:

cranberrylane.com

brambleberry.com

elementsbathandbody.com

soapmaking.com

Chapter 4: Soap Making Equipment

Basic Soap Making Equipment

Most soap making equipment may be found in the kitchen. You may even repurpose existing materials to create soap making equipment. You do not need to have an additional budget for it. But, if you intend to make your own soap kitchen, you may want to invest in the following equipment:

1. Stainless steel pots. You should have at least one 4-liter pot. You may use bigger pots if you want to produce more.

2. Plastic bowls, pitchers or buckets. Pitchers are more preferred than bowls. These will be used for mixing the ingredients. It will be easier to pour the mixtures if the mixing container has a nozzle. Have at least one 4-liter container,

2 2-liter containers, and 2 1-liter containers.

3. Spatulas. Rubber and/or silicone spatulas are preferred. They can be used to mix the mixture. If you have the budget for a hand mixer, it may come in handy, especially with making big batches.

4. Measuring cups and spoons. The lye to oil ratio to be used for each soap recipe should be measured accurately. If the lye is less, the stage of saponification may fail. If the lye is more, the soap may damage the skin.

5. Weighing scale. This is useful when you are using crystallized lye. It is also necessary for measuring other materials, like oatmeal and other extracts.

6. Plastic or wooden molds. This is for molding the soap. There are plastic molds that are flexible, which makes it easier to remove the soap. You

may use baking loaf pans and just slice the soap into smaller or thinner shapes.

7. Wool blankets. This will be used to insulate the soap.

8. Small Sprayer. It will be used to spray alcohol on the soap to reduce the bubbling during the pouring of the mixture.

9. Knives. These will be used to cut the soap. If you want cleaner edges for your soap, you may opt to buy a soap cutter.

10. Cooking or Candy Thermometer. You should invest in these if you intend to make soap using the hot process.

Safety Equipment

Lye is a corrosive material. If it encounters your skin, it may burn your skin and cause injury, especially if it has been dissolved in liquid. It also has a smelly fume that may make you feel nauseated for some time. The use of lye in soap making poses a danger to you and to the people in your home who may mistake lye as other liquid or crystals used in cooking. When storing and using lye, you need to have safety equipment to protect your skin from its effects.

Another safety concern is the use of fire. You may need to cook some ingredients or melt some soap using fire. This may start a fire causing an accident.

Below is a list of safety equipment you may need when making soap:

1. Apron. Use a heavy-duty plastic apron and not the kind you use in cooking. This will protect you from any accidental splashes of the lye-oil solution during mixing.

2. Gloves. These are necessary, especially in measuring or using the lye solutions. You may use rubber gloves during mixing, but you may use the thin cellophane

gloves when cutting the soap. Even though you might find gloves too cumbersome; they are still highly recommended to use. In case lye still gets on your hands, immediately wash your hands under running water, after that, you can also rinse with some vinegar which, as an acid, should neutralize any remaining lye that is left.

3. Goggles. You need to protect your eyes from accidental splashes. Lye solution accidents may result in blindness if you are not careful. In case some of the lye splatters and hits your eyeball, flush your eye for about 15 minutes under running water and go to the emergency room where the doctor should check if there is any remaining lye in your eye.

4. Small fire extinguishers. There are small fire extinguishers which you can buy at the store. It would be helpful to have one under your table when making soap.

5. Masks. You only need to wear masks during the early stage of soap making. As mentioned above, the lye fumes may make you feel dizzy for a while. Wearing masks may help you avoid this, but even just in case you feel a little dizzy after handling lye, don't worry too much, usual lye caused dizziness should stop in 10- 15 minutes.

Safety Rules When Making Soaps

To avoid accidents, you may consider following these safety rules when making soaps:

1. Always wear your safety gear.

2. Do not cook the soap base with your small children. Their curiosity about the process may cause accidents in your kitchen.

3. After measuring the lye, keep the remaining lye in a safe place and far from the reach of children. The shorter the

exposure of the lye chemical on your table, the lower the risk of lye solution accidents.

4. Label your oils and your chemicals. This is necessary if you are using your kitchen in making soap. You may confuse the lye powder with salt or sugar.

5. Clean your equipment and ingredients after soap making. Do not leave your used equipment and ingredients on your work table. Your pet or child may be curious and accidentally play with them.

Chapter 5: Soap Making - The Basics

Soap is a very basic and important commodity today. It is used to clean your body, and sanitize objects that are considered "dirty".

History has been a bit vague when it comes to the origin of the soap. One legend has it that rain water from the slopes of Mount Sapo washed animal tallow and ash onto the clay soil of the banks of Tiber. People then used this material to clean textile. But this legend is very questionable since nobody knows where Mount Sapo actually is.

There are basically two ways to create soap. The first process is the "Melt and Pour" while the second one is the "Cold Process". Both techniques speak for themselves. The only problem now is how to do it exactly.

Today, soap is being manufactured by large companies promoting anti bacterial and skin whitening slogans that accompany their products. Smaller soap makers and soap enthusiasts label their soap with healing qualities. A particular example for this type would be a soap that actually heals your soul. But no matter how the soap is packaged or marketed, they are all made of the same basic ingredients.

Water, lye, and oil are what you basically need for creating soap. For the "Melt and Pour" process, water and lye are heated to a certain temperature, then allowed to cool, adding the oil later after the solution has cooled enough. As for the "Cold Process" of creating soap, the basic instructions would be to combine the water and lye, and stir vigorously. Let it stand for a couple of minutes then add your oil and stir vigorously again before pouring the trace products onto your mold.

HOW TO CREATE YOUR OWN SOAP MAKING RECIPE

Once you've mastered the basics of soap making, it's fun to create your own recipes.

First, you have to decide what method of soap making you're going to make. Are you going to use the cold process method (with lye), the rebatched/handmilled method or the melt and pour method?

Next, what kind of soap do you want to make? For example, prettily molded hand soap or moisturizing soap to use in the bath or shower?

Are you going to superfat your soap? Superfatting is when you add additional fatty oils after saponification to make a richer, creamier soap. There are all kinds of different oils you can use in superfatting, including shea butter and cocoa butter.

What color do you want your soap? What do you want your soap to smell like? What shape and size mold do you want to use? These are important questions to consider.

Do you want to include additives such as oatmeal, flower petals or glitter?

Once you've carefully crafted your own recipe and written instructions, have all the ingredients and equipment necessary, it's time to start making your soap.

Now don't forget you have to allow time for the soap to set and cure. If you're making cold process soap, this takes two weeks. On the other hand, making soap using the melt and pour method only takes a few hours to set, even less if you put it in the refrigerator!

If you plan on giving your soap to friends and family, they're sure to be impressed by the fact that you made the soap yourself, using your own recipe! If you know they like a specific scent, shapes or colors, you can tailor make the soap to their liking, e.g., making lavender seashells for someone who likes seashells and lavender fragrance.

It's really satisfying to make soap using your own recipe. Once you've mastered the art of soap making, or even enjoying the process of mastering it, you may find it hard to stop!

How to Make Your Own Soap

There are various methods and many instructions on how to make your own soap, including;

Cold process method - this is for people who want make soap from scratch, and uses a mixture of lye, water, animal or vegetable fats and oils to produce the soap. It is a fairly easy method to learn, but is quite time consuming and involves handling caustic lye solutions.

Hot process method - similar to the cold process, using heat to speed up the soap making task. The advantage of the hot process is that the soap can be used more or less straight away. If you want to find out how to make your own soap using this method, it's a good idea to start with the cold process first.

Rebatching method - this is a really easy way to learn to how to make your own soap, as it uses melted soap scraps as a base for creating soap bars.

Melt and pour method - similar to rebatching, the melt and pour type of soap making is the easiest way for beginners to learn how to make your own soap without having to deal with lye mixing. The advantage of melt and pour over rebatching is that you use a pre-made natural soap base and add coloring, fragrance and even texture to create your own soap products.

Producing natural, handcrafted soap bars is a great way of making beautiful gifts for your mother, grandmother or any of your female friends or family, once you know how. To make your own soap gifts, the melt and pour method is the best way to do this, as you have control over the ingredients you want to use. Start learning how to make your own soap by using a simple recipe at first, adding just one or two scented oils to ensure that your soap fragrance is not too overpowering. Once you have practiced with a few different aromatherapy or fragrance oils, you could try using colors to make your own soap more appealing to the eye.

THE SOAP MAKING SUPPLIES YOU NEED AND THEIR IMPORTANCE

Soap making enthusiasts have been increasing in numbers over the years. If you just learned about this through the internet or through friends I would gladly say that you should try it. You will be amazed how wonderful and rewarding soap making can be. You do not only need to know the process but also what soap making supply you need.

The supplies you need are the basic ingredients you need in making them. Therefore it is important to be acquainted with the ingredients and learn about its characteristics and functions. You need soap making supplies like lye, fragrance oils, basic oils, equipments and molds.

I will share to you the basic supplies you need:

1. Safety devices - you will need rubber gloves and goggles to protect your skin & eyes from burns. This is the very first thing you need before starting the process even in preparation time.

2. Weighing scale - you need a weighing scale that shows measurements in grams and in ounces. Soap making requires

accuracy in measuring ingredients, therefore it is vital to have one.

3. Containers - the containers you need are not just any container, it should be heat resistant. Have a three-quarter size or bigger depending on your need.

4. Stainless pots - Use only large stainless pots when mixing the lye, basic oils or fats and fragrance oils.

5. Stainless sauce pans - Basically a three-quart stainless sauce pan is used for heating the solid ingredients oils, fats and additives.

6. Silicone Utensils - Use only this type of utensil when mixing your ingredients or any other soap solutions. Wood on the other hand will tend to corrode when it comes in contact with lye and breaks which in the long run makes it expensive because you need to repurchase again. That is why I highly recommend the use of silicone utensils.

7. Thermometers - You need this in measuring lye and oil temperatures.

8. Soap molds - you can be creative when choosing your soap molds. You can buy or make your own soap whichever you want as long as it is suitable with the kind of soap you are making. What is important is to determine how often you are going to use your mold. If you are making soaps only for your family then you can use any soap molds. But if you are planning to make soap making a business, I suggest you buy quality molds available in reputable stores.

9. Wax Paper - you need to place wax paper in your molds for ease of removing your soap bars from its mold and to cover your finished products to preserve heat from dispersing so fast. You may buy any brand of wax paper in the supermarket.

10. Tapes - this is used to keep wax paper in place.

11. Soap cutter - this are optional soap equipment. If you are only making soaps for the family, you may use kitchen knife instead. But if you are cutting soap for selling purposes then a soap cutter is required for finer and clean edges.

12. Fragrance oils and other additives - These are optional as well. If you want your soap to have additives like essential oils or scents then you just buy the particular oil you want. But of course you need to follow precautionary steps, use oils that are compatible with your other ingredients and that blends well with an organic soap making supply.

Now, you are ready to start your newly found hobby and enjoy experimenting with your own ingredients. Have a wonderful time going through the process.

Chapter 6: What Kind Of "Soapie" Are You?

Making soap is an ancient tradition and has been around for many centuries. Who would have thought that they were making soap from plant parts and ash in ancient Roman times? Soap used to solely be a luxury item but now it serves so many purposes:

as a crucial component in the fight against disease and especially to fight bacteria in hospitals

for basic cleanliness

as a luxury item

as a gift

as a fragrance in a drawer

Its value should never be underestimated. Nowadays, because we use different ones for different reasons, smells, designs and even shapes have come a long way in the making of the humble bar of soap.It is because of the myriad ways to make soap and present it and because of innovative new products, soap-making is undergoing a revival and is, once again, becoming a popular industry for those who want to return to a more traditional style.

As soap has been a long- time, favourite gift for family, it represents the perfect way to give a very personalized gift to a friend or family member on special occasions. You can opt for the simple process of "melt and pour" soap or the more involved "cold" process.

Melt and pour means you do not have to make the soap yourself and you can buy a plain, ready-made bar. With the "cold" process, you need to take all the safety precautions and understand the quantities in order to make the perfect soap bar.

It all depends on what kind of soap you prefer or what soap you think is best for the person you are making it for.

So, what kind of soap person are you? And, what kind of soap person is the recipient of your batch of soap? There are indeed different categories of "soap people."

We have the suburban soapies

The posh soapies

The contemporary soapies

The bohemian soapies

The tell-it-like-it-is soapies

The traditional soapies

The nature lover soapies

The sweet-sweet soapies

The super-smelly soapies

In defining your "soapie" style, ask yourself if you like the lavenders, the basil, the potpourri, the sanitized smell, the baby smell, the oaky smell, the smell to clear the sinuses, the sweet smell or perhaps a range of smells depending on its intended use. You can then decide which oils and fragrances to add to your soap.

Talking about soapies...Have you ever wondered why we call the typical TV serial a "soapie?" Speculative answers abound as people tend to think that it is because "soapies" are usually microcosms of daily life and mundane activities – like washing.

However, although they have their origins surrounding the housewife, they have received this name because of the main sponsors of these shows when they were first aired in the 1970s and 1980s.

Of course housewives need to do a lot of cleaning and, around midday, they would have had their lunch break and, often, turned on the TV. Apologies to any housewives out there; this is not meant to stereotype you, it is just the facts surrounding the thinking of the sponsors at the time when "soapies" were popularized.

So, you've guessed it, the manufacturers of detergents and soaps used the TV breaks to advertise their products so it meant that they were the main sponsors. Interesting, don't you think?

Chapter 7: History Of Soap

What are Soaps?

As humans, we have been told all of our life that it is important to use soap after using the restroom, before eating, etc. Has it ever crossed your mind if this really works? Or better yet, why it works? Before answering these questions, it is imperative first to ask ourselves. What is the meaning of dirty? What are we using soap to clean? There are examples such as mud/dust on the skin or dried food burnt onto dishes; the examples on this list go on and on, but all these examples of cleaning have something in common oil is a major player. Water finds it hard to clean off dirt/grime, and this is simply due to the fact that water molecules are more attracted to one another, thus reducing its affinity to oil. As a result of this, water and oil do not mix. This is something we all have been taught in elementary school, with several experiments. The molecules present in the oil are large and non-polar as opposed to the water that is composed of very polar molecules; thus, the two cannot bond together. This explains why it is near impossible to use just water to clean off dirt on your hands. Or, using only water to clean a greasy dish, the water just bounces off without removing the grimes because the oily molecules cannot bond with water. Soap is not a new invention by modern-day humans, ancient people already figured out how to make substances that are soap-like materials that settled the raging battle between water and oil thousands of years ago, thus, creating soap.

In recent years, soap production is a simple industrial business; now, soaps are produced with more sophistication, and they smell way better now. Nonetheless, we still get the same result from both ancient soaps and modern ones. Soap works by separating the large oil particles into smaller drops, therefore, making it possible to mix with water. Soap is able to end the deep hatred between oil and water due to a simple quality it possesses, the particles of soap have two different ends. There is a hydrophilic end, and this is the part of the soap molecule that likes water. This part of the soap is ready to mix with water due to its ionic nature. The other end is referred to as the hydrophobic end that refuses to mix with water as such it is repelled by it. Since the molecules of soap have both polar and non-polar properties, the soap acts as an emulsifier that is capable of bridging the gap between two unmixable liquids. When water and soap are mixed, the molecules of the soap place themselves into tiny clusters or micelles. As such, the parts of the soap that love water points out, while the parts that hate water come together on the inside, due to the repulsion from water. These hydrophobic parts collect the oil particles in the centre, trapping the oil in the soap and when this is washed off with water, the hydrophilic parts attract water, taking away both the soap and the grime attached to the soap.

History of Soap.

The process of soap making goes back thousands of years, and archaeologists have since discovered actual scientific evidence that the Mesopotamian civilization in 3200 BC actually used a mixture of tree ash and animal fats to manufacture a simple soap. Although there are different claims from several quarters on the civilization that actually first created soap, it is impossible to deny the existence of soap during ancestral times, and it is very much around now – Yes! Soap is basically meant for cleaning dirt. It is quite impossible to say that some kind of washing did not happen before the era of soap commercialization. However, it is still difficult to pinpoint the exact era when soap was first created. Clay pots filled with materials that looked like soap-material were uncovered during the Babylon era (2800 BC), but it remains unclear maybe it is actually soap or not; as it was also used as a hair styling product. There is a popular opinion that the Egyptians were the first set of humans that bathed regularly. Thankfully, this perception was widely accepted. The soap recipe of the Egyptians was discovered on a medical document that is referred to as Ebers-Papyrus (1500 BC). This recipe was used for many purposes, such as personal cleansing and treatment for skin diseases.

Apart from the Egyptians and the Mesopotamians, the Greeks also used a type of soap for cleaning their dishes and the statues of their Gods. This soap was manufactured by combining common ashes and lye. However, the Egyptians did not use soap whenever they bathe. Instead, they use items like pumice and clay while they used oil to scent themselves. Soap is an integral part of human life when it comes to cleaning and washing stuff. All widely practised religions, consider cleanliness as next to godliness. These religions usually set certain instructions and guidelines when it comes to the maintenance of cleanliness in all sacred places. Cleanliness sometimes signifies the importance of soul and body; it has also been a part of prayer. For instance, when describing Herodotus (485-425 BCE), there was a detailed explanation of the purification process and what was expected of the priest- physicians in the Temple that is called Amun at Kamak in Egypt when King Ramses was ruling between 1113-1085 BCE: "Bathe in cold water twice a day and twice a night and cleansed mouth with natron" Natron is combination of sodium carbonate and sodium bicarbonate. These rituals were carried out regularly, as they indicate rejuvenation and rebirth. In the wild, animals and birds keep themselves clean regularly in different ways. Birds bathe in water and use their beaks to clean their feathers. Cats, Dogs, and other wild animals lick their bodies to keep them clean.

The Pre-soap Era

In the olden days, several methods were utilized or used for cleanliness by humans from different parts of the globe. The Neolithic people used flint scrapers to clean their body. Before the period of Pliny, the Elder (23-79 CE), the Romans and Greeks did not use soap, but they used the heat generated by vapour baths and by scrubbing with skin scrappers made from ivory, bone, or metal. Through the methods, they were able to accomplish the vital cleaning of their bodies. Ancient Egyptians used soda for cleansing, and they also utilized soda for the transformation of a diseased skin to healthy skin. Before the advent of Christianity, olive oil was used by people when anointing their bodies, and they also cleaned their skin with Fuller's earth and plant ashes. Plant ashes were used as soap substitutes or soap by several civilizations. Soaps were produced from plant derivatives during the biblical period. Most of the plants' derivatives used during this period can be found in the salty regions of Arabia and contained soda and potash majorly. Some of the soap producing plants include – Syrian ahala, Akkadian uhulu, and Arabic gasul. Ashleg was employed for washing materials in the rabbinical literature. In other areas such as the Indian subcontinent and in Chile, Peru, and Angola, clay and plant ashes were widely used as soap, and it is still in use in some places in recent years. During the recent Angolan civil war that spanned twenty years, several individuals used different plants due to the scarcity of commercial soaps.

The Origin of the Word "Soap"

Although it is not clear where the word "soap" originated from, several legends have documented the origin of the word. According to one of these manuscripts, soap- production accidentally started close to 3000 years ago on Mount Sapo, near Rome. Animals provided by the peasants were sacrificed and burned to the gods on Mount Sapo. Ashes of the altar fires and fats from the burned animals mixed over time. The mixture eventually made its way downhill over the clay soil. People that visited the temple found out that the mixture of slippery clay aided the cleaning and washing of clothes. In Gaul, a man once dressed his hair with beech tree ashes and goat oil. He later got caught in the rain, the man he noticed the formation of lather in his hair. The English word "soap" was derived from the Latin word "sapo". "Soap" as a word is a Teutonic contribution, and it is gotten from the Anglo-Saxon "sape" and the Middle English "sope." Although different languages have different terms and pronunciation when it comes to soap. The term "detergent" is a descriptive word gotten from the Latin word "detergee", which means clean or wipe. The word detergent most of the time refers to synthetic soap.

Early Soap-making

Sumerian clay tablets that date back to the third millennium BCE in Boghszkoi the capital of Hittite gave the earliest written account of soap production and usage. "With water, I bathed myself, with soda I cleansed my- self, with oil from the basin I beautified myself." During an archaeological expedition in the ancient city of Babylon from the Ur dynasty, an excavated Sumerian clay cylinder found during the excavation of the city contained a soap production process that involves the use of alkali, oil, and water. According to Pliny, the Elder - Phoenicians discovered soap production in 600 BCE. In his classic description, Pliny stated the process of making soap from the fats of goats and the ashes of beech trees.

The Graeco-Roman Period

The Romans and Greeks used flours of lentils and oils as substitutes for real soaps. They used soaps as hair pomade instead of utilizing them for the cleaning of their bodies. Romans picked up the soap making process and the use of soap either from the Celts or ancient Mediterranean peoples. The Celts made soap from plant ashes and animal fat and referred to the product as "saipo". In the 8th century CE, an Arab warrior Jabir Ibn Hayyan (Gaber), talked about using soap as a cleansing agent on separate instances. Soap was produced from woods ashes and mutton tallow during the Roman period, and a type of rough soap was made in France about 100 CE. Between 700-800 CE, soap production became a craft industry in Spain and Italy. The original Castile soap was produced from wood ashes, perfumes, and olive oil during this era in Spain.

The Medieval Period and Later

During the middle ages, Marseilles became the first soap producing city in Europe, followed by Genoa, and Venice soon followed suit. Soap was manufactured in Germany, but it was not used widely as a cleaning agent. The first soap production in England start in Bristol around 1200AD, and over the course of the next 200 years, a small community was created around the neighbourhood of Cheapside in London basically for soap production. During this period, people making soap had to pay taxes on soaps they manufactured. By the start of the Napoleonic Wars, the levy on soap production has increased significantly, and it maintained the status quo until it was stopped in 1853. For many years, the production of soap was majorly small-scale with ingredients such as plant ashes with carbonate dispersed into the water; fat was also included after a period of time. Ashes were used to boil this mixture until the water evaporates. A slow chemical reaction happens during this process due to the mixture of fatty acid with alkali carbonates of the plant ashes, leading to the formation of soap. This reaction is widely referred to as saponification. The process was employed until the end of the Middle Ages when slaked lime was introduced. Over time, soap production became a craft in Europe in the seventh century. There was the establishment of European soap making guilds. These guilds remained a secret, and each sect guarded their trade secrets very closely. The European soap making guilds were the first group of people that fragranced their soaps.

Within a short period of time, trees became a vital raw material for the production of soap. This is due to the fact that soil type played a huge role when it comes to the establishment of soap plants. Marseilles in France is widely regarded as the first location of the pioneer soap plants. The city had an amazing soil that is quite productive for vegetable sodas and olive trees. Before this, vegetable soda and olive tree oil were brought in from overseas. Spain and Italy were the major importers. Soap producing plants became very popular and different plants began to spring up in both countries consecutively. This unannounced battle for supremacy between the two nations continued until the twelfth century when France took over the reins with the production of olive oil soap as opposed to other soaps that were produced with different materials. From that point, the production of soap on a large scale continued to experience a meteoric rise. King James, I monopolized soap producers for $100,000 per annum and special treatment in 1622. This continued deep into the 19th century. Up until this period time, every soap was heavily taxed due to the fact that it is seen as a luxury item. This tax made it near impossible for a common man to have access to soap, thus putting a stop to the cleanliness level of the commoners. The masses only experienced good skin health and cleanliness when the high tax was scrapped.

Modem Soap Manufacturing

Towards the end of the 18th century, unfolding events led to the evolution of the handcrafted soap production to industrial-level production. The Government of France in 1775 via the Academy of Science, announced a reward for the pioneer production of an acceptable industrial process for the conversion of sodium chloride into sodium carbonate. This feat was achieved by Nicolas Le Blanc in 1790 when he produced soda ash from ordinary table salt, and he was given the prize. Nicholas Le Blanc was the first name to be tied to soap since he was the first person to discover a cheap method extracting soda from table salt. This new type of soap production quickly spread like wildfire and with time, more discoveries and innovations were achieved to make soap production easier. During this period, soaps also continued to experience more usage and popularity among the populace.

Claude Berthollet found out the bleaching power of chlorine which was first produced by Carl Wilhelm Scheele in 1774, and Charles Tennant in 1799 produced bleaching powder by absorbing chlorine in lime. The first settler in North America used homemade soap. They produced soap through their native soap production process. By adding boiling water to plant ashes in bids to make potash and boiling it in animal fat, they produced soap. Eugene-Michel Chevreul in 1811 became the next standout name in the history of soap production when he determined the exact amount of glycerin, animal fat, and fatty acids that were needed for the production of quality soap. Prior to his discovery, the recipes used for soap production was based on a guess of ingredient measurements. This was yet another groundbreaking discovery that helped shaped the popularity of soap in human history. Soap manufacturing on a large scale basis started in North America in the 19th century when wasted fats were gathered from villages. By the 1850s, soap production became one of America's fastest-growing sectors, and it was also during this period that soap became a necessity as opposed to the previous perception that classified it as a luxury.

With all of the new discoveries and inventions that are currently happening in the world of soap, production diversified into the making of soap varieties and suppliers. Soap was made in the open in big kettles. This mixture was then poured into huge wooden boxes and then cut into bars which are then sold from door to door. Sulfonated castor oil that is referred to as turkey red oil is the first synthetic surfactant and it was introduced as a cleanser in 1851. German scientist- Fritz Gunther is known for the creation of synthetic detergent in 1916. The detergent he produced was quite rough and harsh; thus, it was used mainly for industrial purposes. The first household detergent was produced by Proctor & Gamble in 1933. The production of a milder soap means there was a distinction between detergent for clothes and body soap. Soap making did not stop there, in 1938, the Food, Drug, and Cosmetic Act was passed. This act gave soap producers the liberty to produce different types of soap, and this made soaps more regulated like what is obtainable in the present day.

Various Types of Soap

Detergents and soaps are the potassium or sodium salts of long-chain fatty acids employed for cleaning purposes and excipient in the production of suppositories and pills. In history, soap is referred to as "sapo durus" ("hard soap"), "sapo mollis" ("soft soap"), and "sapo vividen" ("green soap"). The main ingredient of hard soap or "sapo durus" is soda, and this soap is majorly greyish-white in colour when it becomes dry and cold. It is used majorly for external cleaning purposes. Softsoap or "sapo mollis" resembles jelly or honey, and it is usually scentless, yellowish and translucent, and it will readily turn soluble in rectified spirit. The major ingredients are potash and olive oil. Softsoap, in a dose of 5 to 20gm, was utilized as an antacid. Green soap is a special type of soft soap that is used majorly for treating seborrheic dermatitis of the scalp. There are several types of soaps for different purposes. Medicated soaps are composed of tar, phenol, glycerin, and several oils. Liquid soaps usually contain potassium salts of fatty acids of olive, coconut, soybean, castor oil, or cottonseed. Cake or solid soaps are sodium salts of fatty acid, and sometimes potassium salts are also present.

Medical Uses of Soap

When checking out history, soap was also used as a medicinal agent in different kinds of literature on separate occasions. Claudius Galen (130-200 CE) talked about the medical and skin cleansing properties of soap. Ferdinand von Hebra (1816-1880) also used soap for the treatment of several skin problems such as psoriasis, scabies, psoriasis, herpes tonsurans and tinea versicolor. When it comes to the treatment of psoriasis, Hebra told his patients to "make a sort of plaster by spreading soft soap, like an ointment, over pieces of flannel, and apply these to the spots affected, until they soften the epidermis and remove masses of scale." Hebra also advised people to use "spiritus saponatous alkalinus" for the treatment of milia. In Europe during the 19th Century, a process referred to as "soap cure" was used regularly to treat skin diseases. Superfatted soap (basic soap) was introduced for skin treatment uses by Paul Gerson Unna (1850-1929) of Hamburg. Soap was also used to treatment of acne vulgaris, tinea and freckle versicolor, and other mycotic conditions. Charles J. White (1869-1964) from Boston used Ivory soap and Castile for the treatment of acne. A look at the history of soap shows the continuous effort of humans to maintain hygiene. The production of different kinds of agents frequently parallels our perception of cosmetics and chemicals.

Chapter 8: Hand Sanitizer

1.1 Important facts to know about Hand sanitizer

There is a high demand for hand sanitizer during this period, due to the fast spread of the virus. The best defense against contracting any kind of virus consists of firstly maintaining high standard hygiene, by washing hands regularly since this simple action can drastically reduce the bacterial load rested on the hands' skin. It is important to keep in mind that the homemade sanitizer is to be used as a substitution of water and soap in case the latter is not accessible.

Hand sanitizer is a liquid or gel generally used to decrease infectious agents on the hands, in the healthcare setting, having more effect on killing microorganisms. Since the first humans started to live in modern homes, as we conceived today, to be attentive to cleanliness has been a priority. Also the fact of moving entire families or groups of people in secure homes, was an idea to escape from the external danger and gain protection in protected houses. The objective was to protect themselves from animals, enemy attacks, negative weather conditions and last but not least from the virus and bacteria.

Antoni Van Leeuwenhoek was the first one who discovered the bacteria, and understood that it could infect the people and the enormous gravity that it could be spread from person to person. Going back with the ages, we can know that the first instruments invented by our ancients, were composed of brooms and brushes, used from cleaning. The constant need to live in acceptable hygienic conditions is fundamental in our life, and later on, the rise of the industrial revolution, the mechanization brought high improvements to tools: technology and mechanics entered in our homes, as also professional cleaning stuff evolved too.

With the economical boom, which began in 1950, mostly the USA had a rise in almost all the sectors, including unneeded goods and electro domestics. This started a period called "The Good Life", which marked an incredible expansion of the entire economy, including the production of manufacturing, plastic and electronics. Another consequence of this boom was the expansion of the housing sector and marriages. American society started to be considered a consumerist country, and the consumption became a habit for the community to copy. Homes, from places where to sleep after work, became part of the people community. A big part of the family budget was allocated to make them new and comfortable, creating nests of love.

Regarding the origin, the gel-based hand sanitizer was invented in 1966 and it was originally only used in sanatorium, hospices, hospitals and medical settings. The product started to be used for home and personal use until the 1980s and 1990s. In 1966 however, a nursing student named Lupe Hernandez from Bakersfield, California, found out that alcohol could be delivered in a gel: thus discovering hand sanitizer. Originally it was only used in hospital settings until it became commercialized by companies like Purell and Gojo in 1988.

1.2 Why is it important to clean your hands properly?

Washing your hands is the best way to protect yourself, your family and your community. It is very safe to wash your hands if you cough or blow your nose, when you make or eat food when you touch animals and you play with them, after using the toilet, when you play and do sport outdoor.

Hand hygiene is an essential practice to protect yourself against many diseases and infections. Indeed, regular hand washing is a simple, quick and effective way to prevent the spread of viruses and bacteria and thus the transmission of infectious diseases.

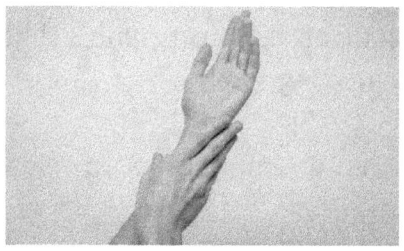

The risk of contamination is also much higher in collective environments (public transport, public places, etc.) where access to a water point is not always possible. Therefore, to reduce any risk of transmission or infection, the use of a sanitizer solution is recommended.

Germs can spread when:

You touch your eyes, nose, and mouth with your hands

You touch the food with unwashed hands

You touch surfaces or objects

You blow your nose, and sneeze and after you touch the other people's hands.

1.3 How should you wash your hands?

Washing your hands is a key part of preventing the spread of viruses. We can tell you the exact way to wash them. Wet your hands with clean water that could be warm or cold. When you are in front of your sink, rotate off the tap, and apply soap. Flap your hands by rubbing them together with the soap. Be sure to foam the back of your hands, among your fingers, and above your nails

Clean your hands for at least 20 seconds. You can sing your favorite song or the national hymn of your country! Wash your hands for the duration of the song and continue under running water and then use a clean wipe or a paper towel to turn off the faucet, and then throw it away.

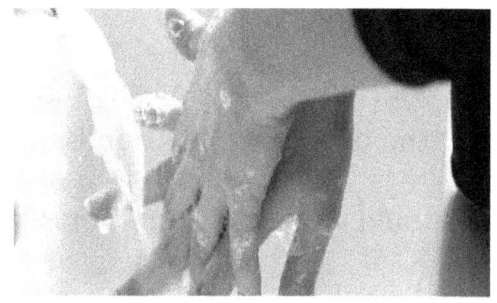

1.4 Which kind of germs the hand sanitizer kills?

The transmission of a virus can be done also from a contaminated surface. The virus stays on it for up to 20 minutes. Some viruses, like Salmonella and Coli, can live up two hours on surfaces. A temperature of 140 degrees of the water can kill the virus. Germs are also transmitted from unclean hands to food by an infected person who touches the food and didn't wash their hands after using the toilet. It is known that touching and eating food with dirty hands is not good for our body, but we know what happens if we do it. 15-30% of viral and bacterial infections are transmitted by the main vehicle of contagion, our hands, and this can be prevented by observing careful hygiene.

The hands are also in constant contact with our mouth and during the day they touch many contaminated surfaces, such as cell phones, shared keyboards, external surfaces to which everyone has contact, especially children who, unaware of bacteria and contaminations, put everything in their mouth regardless of the consequences.

Easy to take everywhere with you and practical to use, these products with bactericidal, virucidal and fungicidal properties allow you to quickly disinfect your hands wherever you are. This makes them a good alternative to conventional hand washing.

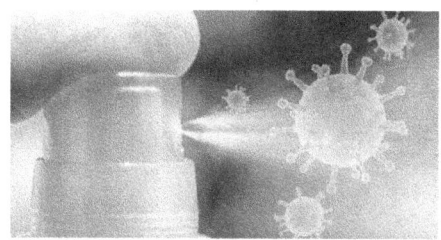

1.5 Which ingredients do you need to make your homemade hand sanitizer?

¾ cup of isopropyl or rubbing alcohol (99 percent alcohol volume)

¼ cup of aloe Vera gel

10 drops of essential oil, such as tea tree oil or lavender oil, or you can use lemon juice instead.

Nitrile gloves so you don't burn your hands when making the hand sanitizer.

The role of the essential oils is important for the fragrance of the mix. Then your sanitizer will be also a pleasure for you if you are used to the smell, and on the other hand, those not expensive products.

1.5.1 #Alcohol

Isopropyl alcohol is a colorless, flammable chemical compound (chemical formula $CH_3CHOHCH_3$) with a strong odor. Be careful not to use any other types of alcohol like methanol, butanol, as they are toxic.

Isopropyl alcohol is miscible in water, ethanol, ether and chloroform. It is able to dissolve ethyl cellulose, polyvinyl butyral, many oils, alkaloids, gums and natural resins. Unlike ethanol or methanol, isopropyl alcohol is not miscible with saline solutions and can be separated from aqueous solutions by adding a salt such as sodium chloride. The process is called salting out and allows to concentrate isopropyl alcohol in a distinct phase. You can find this product in pharmacies, drugstores or also on Amazon.

1.5.2 #Aloe Vera

You need to mix the isopropyl alcohol with another element; on its own it will burn your hands. The ideal solution is aloe Vera gel as it acts as a natural moisturizer. Aloe Vera is a medicinal plant. It has been used to treat various health conditions, centuries ago.

It's usually also safe to use Vera directly from the plant. Recently you can enjoy it in gel form. Aloe Vera creams, gels, and ointments contain the clear gel found in aloe Vera leaves. These products can be used usually to treat various skin conditions. Aloe is sold in capsule or liquid form to take internally to promote health and well-being. In Egypt, 6,000 years ago, Aloe Vera was considered the plant of immortality, also used during funerals or as a gift to pharaohs.

1.5.3 #Essential oils to use

Tea tree oil

Tea tree oil is an essential oil that can be used for several purposes, including keeping skin, hair, and nails healthy. Tea tree oil has been used as traditional medicine by Aborigines for centuries. These native Australians squeeze tea tree leaves to extract the oil, which is then inhaled to treat coughs and colds or applied directly to the skin for healing.

Lavender oil

Lavender oil - or, more precisely, lavender essential oil - is a compound obtained from the flowering tops of Lavandula angustifolia, a plant belonging to the Labiatae family.

Lavender oil has numerous properties, which make it useful in the external treatment of several ailments. In particular, this oil is widely used in the field of aromatherapy, where it is renowned for its calming and relaxing properties.

Several studies have confirmed that lavender essential oil has a moderate antibacterial activity (albeit lower than that possessed by other oils, such as, for example, rosemary essential oil), associated with an interesting antifungal activity.

Lavander essential oil is capable of exerting a depressive action on the central nervous system, which is also carried out by simply inhaling the product.

Lavender oil is attributed with interesting anti-inflammatory properties, which seem to be exercised through the inhibition of the activity of phospholipase C. Furthermore, a study has shown that lavender essential oil is also able to exert an antinociceptive action.

Lemon juice

Lemons are high in vitamin C, fiber, and various beneficial plant compounds. These nutrients are responsible for several health benefits. It has antioxidant properties due to the citric acid contained in it. This precious juice also has antioxidant properties. And there is much more. As it is known, lemon juice contains significant quantities of vitamin C (100 grams bring more than 100% of the daily dose), powerful antioxidant, a valid ally of our immune defenses and in the absorption of iron. As if it were a magic potion, here are some of the numerous benefits made from cheap and easily available lemon juice (more than that!):it promotes digestion; stimulates the function of the liver and intestines; used together with baking soda, it helps whiten your teeth; soothes sunburn and insect bites; antiseptic, it works well as a first intervention disinfectant; soothing for the feet, if used for foot baths; on the skin, excellent as anti-acne, anti-eczema and against "age spots".

According to US scientific studies, lemon is an excellent support for the elimination of kidney stones, and it is believed to have positive effects also on the control of blood pressure and clotting.

Chapter 9: How To Keep Customers Coming Back

Remember, you're selling an aesthetic experience. Make your logo, the look of your labels and packaging, and the name of your product line resonate with customers seeking a modestly priced luxury experience. One advantage is that the more your customers love your offering the quicker they'll go through it and need more. Make sure you stay in contact with your customers, and that they know how to reach you. Ask all of your customers for email addresses, and get their permission to send out a monthly e-newsletter or catalog. It is important to refrain from irritating anyone with too many salesy emails, but a monthly newsletter can help customers stay up to date with all of the new things you offer. As you grow, you might add a toll-free phone number for orders.

Basic Equipment And Ingredients

If you're like me, once you decide to do something, like making your first batch of soap, you become so excited that you might be tempted to jump in and start making it before you've double checked that you have all the ingredients It's a good idea before you start any session – not just your initial couple of batches – that you have everything you need. And it makes sense to lay them out so you can take inventory of them. If you start on impulse to make a cake or cookies and find that you don't have enough sugar, you can always knock on your neighbor's door to borrow a cup. The chances are good; she'll have it. It's far less likely your neighbor will have a cup of lye for you. The following list contains the basic soapmaking equipment that covers all four processes. Just because it's on the list doesn't necessarily mean you'll need it for the specific technique you're using.

Basic Equipment You Will Need

Ventilated Space

Before you even check out the equipment, you need to find a workspace in your house you can work in – safely. This means that if you've chosen to work with lye – either with the hot or cold process – it means you'll need to be in a well ventilated room. Lye can be corrosive. It's best to take as many precautions as you can when you work with it.

Rubber Gloves, Goggles And Mask

If you choose to work with lye, then you absolutely need the gloves, goggles and the mask. Of course, these are safety precautions, but all it takes is one slip and something volatile may occur. I know that goggles may be expensive, and your budget may be tight, but don't get cheap when it comes to purchasing these safety glasses. You'll want to buy a pair that is much like those used in labs. And, of course, the mask is essential to ensure you're not inhaling lye fumes. This specific equipment especially necessary if you're using either the cold process or the hot process.

Water

Whether you're using the cold process or the hot, you'll find that you'll need distilled water. Distilled water is that which has no minerals or contaminants in it. You may not realize it right now, but you'll notice the difference when you make soap with distilled or tap water. You'll have a need for distilled water for both the hot process and the coal process. You'll also need tap water to wash chemicals and other ingredients from your workspace as well as yourself.

Stainless Steel Pot

If you're using the cold process method, then you'll need one stainless steel pot to dedicate to the use for lye. Double check to ensure that it is indeed stainless steel. You don't want to use aluminum. And don't whatever you do, use this pot for cooking food. Lye has the potential to be dangerous, so it's best to keep it separate from your kitchen equipment.

Stainless Steel Saucepan

You'll need this to heat your additives, including fats and oils. Heat resistant glass containers and measuring cups. Don't think you can slide by using plastic equipment here. Some of the ingredients achieve so hot that it's possible they'll melt plastic.

Measuring Spoons

Now here's a bit of a different warning. When you measure lye, you should use plastic. You're probably surprised by this. But there is a reason for it. There are specific metals that may react with the lye. So, it's best, to dole out the initial lye with plastic spoons. This doesn't mean you should use these for hot solutions, just in case the plastic melts.

Ph Paper

Just in case you're curious, the pH paper is an abbreviation for Phenolphthalein. More commonly, you've probably heard them referred to as litmus strips. You'll use these when you go to check the soap's pH balance. It's highly recommended that you do this when you use the hot process technique.

Pipettes

Technically speaking, these are necessary, but they are just about the easiest tools when you're measuring out small amounts of ingredients. You may find yourself needing to add ingredients in terms of "drops," especially if you're planning on using essential or fragrance oils. These will come in handy using any of the methods.

Digital Scale

When it comes down to it, the digital scale is, without a doubt the most important piece of equipment for the artisan soap making. This may surprise you but consider that these recipes you'll be working with depend on a fairly high degree of accuracy. Specifically, you'll want to purchase a scale that weighs to the tenth of a measurement in ounces and grams. This scale is essential for both the hot and cold processes, and you may even use it for the melt and pour technique as well.

Thermometers

You might want to purchase two of these. These are vital for both the hot and cold processes.

Silicone Spatulas

This particular type of spatula will be essential to help you mix. You definitely don't want to use wood for this portion of the process. You'll discover the need for these, especially, when you're using the hot and cold processes.

Mixing Spoons And Spatulas

You can use wooden or metal spoons and spatulas for anything that doesn't have lye in it. This means these are perfect for the melt and pour technique and when you're re-batching.

Electric Stick Blender

Used in the cold process method, the stick blender can be a valuable tool. Not only that, but this is one piece of equipment you'll be able to use just about anywhere and on anything

Rubbing Alcohol

You should keep a bottle of rubbing alcohol among your basic ingredients as a just-in-case it's a very helpful ingredient to have around. Rubbing alcohol works well at smoothing surfaces on your soap after you've popped any bubbles that may have shown up on your soap. This can occur with either the hot or cold process as well as the melt-and-pour method.

Microwave Or Double Boiler

You may want to use a microwave or a double boiler for the melt-and-pour method to heat the original soap. But I highly recommend you seriously consider using a double boiler. A double boiler is simply a smaller put inside a bigger pot, where the bigger or outer pot holds and warms the water while the inner smaller pot melts the soap base. It is effective, safe and inexpensive to use.

Slow Cooker

Also called by its brand name of Crockpot, you'll only need this if you're making the soap through the hot process technique. Using this appliance accelerates saponification. And don't think you need a slow cooker dedicated to soap making.

Plastic Wrap

You'll need this only if you're using the hot process technique. You'll use this for cover slow cooker after the lye and oils have been mixed.

Knife

What you want to use is a medium-sized knife so you can make clean cuts on your soap and soap bases when you make your product through the melt-and pour method and when you're making re-batches.

Cutting Board

It's good to cut your soap and soap bases on a cutting board, but you don't need an expensive one. You'll be using the using this in the melt-and-pour and rebatching techniques.

Soap Molds

The molds, as you probably know, are used to create the solid shape of your soap. You simply pour the soap into a mold. It's here that it'll harden and take on the shape of the mold. There are a wide variety of molds you can use. By the way, you'll need these for all the processes. You have a choice among four types of molds: plastic, silicone, wooden or paper. Molds made of plastic are less expensive than some categories. But they aren't the easiest to work with. Once the soap hardens, it may not slip out of the mold easily. You really have nothing to learn to give these a try, especially for your first couple of batches. Silicone molds are easy to use and yet quite affordable. Not only this but they're better than the plastic version for getting the hardened soap out of them. But, when you check this out, you'll probably agree that it's not the sturdiest. In some cases, silicone molds have also been known to distort the true shape of the mold and therefore the soap product itself.

Wooden Molds

Never heard of them? If you're not currently making soap, I'm not surprised. They're sturdier than silicone molds and actually provide a more insulated space for the soap. When you use these, you'll have to line them with either wax paper or parchment paper. As you might expect, these are among the costliest molds on the market.

Paper Molds

Paper molds are very inexpensive. No, we're not talking sheets of paper, but rather molds made from paper products, like milk cartons. These molds, obvious, aren't as sturdy as the others, but you'll discover you'll have little trouble taking the hardened soap out of the mold. If bad comes to worse, you can just tear the milk carton away from the soap.

Lining Paper

This paper is needed to line the wooden molds before you pour the liquid into it. If you don't have this, you can use plastic wrap for this as well.

Tape

You'll want the tape to secure that lining paper to the wooden molds.

Soap Cutting Tool

This "cutting tool" is for you to cut the hardened soap into bars. You'll really only need this if you're working with wooden or paper molds.

Chapter 10: Soap Making Tools

Most likely you don't want to mix your soap making tools with general cooking or cleaning tools so you'll likely need to get some new ones to start out. Or better yet recycle some older pots and containers and buy new ones.

It is likely friends and family have utensils and containers they actively want to get rid off so make sure to ask before you spend any money. The only really big difference between hot and cold for the most part is that hot requires you to have a relatively large crock pot or cooking pot.

Staying safe with lye

One of the most important things to make sure is that you are being safe when handling lye and mixing it together with a fat. If you get lye on your skin it can be corrosive and it can't be easily washed off with a little water.

Your skin has a pH of around 7 and if you get something with a very high pH on it will try to equilibrate and raise your skin's pH. Lye eats oils and fats and dissolves proteins on your skin and has a pH of around 14.

If you get lye on your bare skin, you therefore need to bring the pH down quickly. Soap, being derived from lye, actually has a higher pH than your skin and most tap water will be around 7 as well.

An acid like white vinegar with a pH of 2 in theory could be used to neutralize the lye, but you need a lot of vinegar for it to work well and some argue it might cause a hot reaction on your skin.

If you get any on your skin the best option is to remove the clothing it touched and then rinse it with fresh water for several minutes. A small splash on your clothed arm can be dealt with at home with a long shower, but you should seek medical attention for larger splashes or if lye gets near your eyes.

To stop this from happening in the first place make sure you keep safe.

First buy some **rubber gloves**. Don't skimp on these and check to see if the gloves claim to protect against corrosive substances – some cheaper household gloves may not. However, most disposable gloves will do the job.

Then you will need some **safety goggles**. This doesn't mean reading glasses and you'll want more than just swimming goggles. Luckily you can get adequate safety goggles for as little as a $1.

When working try to cover as much skin as possible (long sleeve shirts) and be cautious when dealing with lye. However, don't be so cautious that you end up creating more spills because you were too delicate and kept everything at an arm's length.

Some people like to wear face masks or surgical masks when working with lye. If the area you are in is well ventilated and you make sure to mix the right amount of lye to water you don't need a mask – but you can buy them very cheaply if you feel it is a good idea.

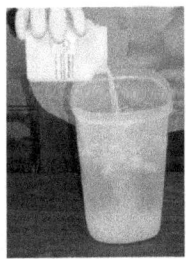

The biggest danger with lye isn't when using it however; it's during storage and cleaning up when you might have ditched the protective gear. Clean down surfaces well with a vinegar-based cleaner and store lye solutions very securely and away from children in a plastic container.

Avoid using metal with lye as it can heat up during the chemical reaction when lye meets water.

Keep your gear on even when handling the soap mixture later (it can still be damaging your skin until the sopanification process is done). Only once it is hardened and you have let it cure will you know it's safe to use.

Soap making equipment

When it comes to general equipment for making soap the first thing to look into is spoons and stirrers. You'll need to mix the lye together with this and also stir in essentials oils and dyes. Make sure they are longer and made of plastic or metal. You will also need a spatula to scrap all the soap mixture into the mould at the end.

When it comes to stirring the lye together with water you'll need a large jug or pitcher made of glass or plastic. Make sure it's more than enough to contain all the water you're going to put in without spilling after mixing.

For measuring out the lye you'll need a good scale that can measure to fairly small and accurate degree. A sensitive digital scale is ideal and you can buy one online for $10 via Amazon. You'll probably put in extra fat to account for the fact your measurement might not be perfect, but you still want to be accurate. Remember to avoid measuring out lye on the same surface you'll be using to measure out food later.

The fats and oils can usually be prepared in your regular pans and dishes (but don't cross-contaminate). When it comes to mixing together the fat and the lye you can use a smaller glass pitcher or a larger metal or glass pot that can easily contain all the ingredients.

Thrift stores will sell older crock pots and pitchers which will be perfectly suited for only a few dollars. Dollar stores will sell plastic pitchers, mixing bowls, spoons, and even plastic spatulas for, well, a dollar each.

To stir together the soap, you will need a stick blender or hand blender. Again these can be bought cheaply and you won't want to be stood there stirring or whisking for ages. These can also be hard to clean so get a new one for your soap making endeavors.

It can be useful to have a thermometer around for both cold and hot process soap, if you are doing hot though you will need one to make sure the temperature is right.

Finally, you will need a mold for your soap. Almost any container can be used to make soap, just ensure that there is enough space for all of the soap mixture and you can easily get the mixture out again.

At this stage the soap is not especially corrosive so you don't have to worry too much about reactions with the remaining lye. Some containers, especially metal containers, are likely to stick to the soap mixture so put down a lining of plastic or parchment to get the soap out later.

You will also need a knife to cut up your block of soap later – but anything can be used to do this as it is just regular soap at that point.

Choosing a mold for your soap

While almost anything can be used as a soap mold there are a few things to consider.

Firstly, how are you going to get your soap out of the mold?

Using a cold process soap you should have a softer soap that you can quite easily take out of the mold but it will still get stuck in more cumbersome containers without the right kind of packaging to help you get it out.

The easiest molds for getting soap out are usually silicon and wooden molds. With silicon you can easily move the sides and plop you soap out. If you can't then it needs to be cured for longer.

With wooden molds you can remove the sides and easily get your soap out.

Plastic and metal molds can be more difficult to get right and will require freezer or wax paper to help you mold out the soap.

Secondly, what shape do you want your soap to be?

Most loaf or square molds will give you just that: square molds. If you want round or circular soap then using a PVC tube can be very useful. Once set you simply freeze the soap and then push it out to be cured.

There are many novelty molds available in the world and you can use Jell-O and cooking molds to make strange and weird looking soaps if you wish (you'll often need to use freezer paper here). The soap bar prevails because it's simple and easy to hold but this is your chance to go wild.

Thirdly, how much do you want to pay?

It is possible to purchase silicon loaf 'tins' from the dollar store that will work well to make soap, but if you want a professional container you will need to pay extra to have perfectly sized soap.

The wooden and silicon trays and molds are not very expensive but considering you can use other molds for free they can add up. If you want to make several types of soap shapes they can really start to add up in price.

Which mold you choose shouldn't make a huge difference to the soap you make – so it is up to you to choose what fits your style. Be careful of treated woods and strange metals. If you want to make patterns in your soap, try to get a deeper mold that will let you work more easily with it.

Choosing a fat for your soap

The biggest question for your soap is which far or oil you are going to use to make a soap. It may seem tempting to just go with a really cheap tallow or vegetable oil, but the idea in soap making is to have a soap you really want to use – not just to save money on soap.

What kind of fats can you use?

The only stipulation when choosing a fat is that it has fatty acid in it – which is true of nearly all animal and plant fats including nut oils.

The big caveat to being able to use any fat is that you need to know how much alkali to use to treat the fat – if you decide to use alligator fat you will struggle to find this information (not to mention you will struggle to get enough alligator fat).

Using the hot process is almost certainly better for soaps with lesser used fats and is why it was favored in the past when they struggled to get the sopanification values and to weigh out the alkali properly.

However, many even seemingly obscure fats have their sopanification values (how much lye or NaOH you need) available including ostrich fat and mink oil. The sopanification values of different animals vary just as much as the values between olive oil and coconut vary so using the value for beef tallow for deer tallow won't work.

Because of this you can use any fat you can get your hands on including human fat and fish oil. If you want, you can even use the cheap vegetable oil you have at home for cooking your dinner.

This brings us to the main point though, choosing your fat is one of the most important elements of making your own soap. It will determine how to use the soap so we'll look at the two biggest things to consider when choosing soap fat: its cost, how hard it is to prepare, its shelf life, and what the kind of soap a fat makes.

The types of oils and fats for soap making

All fats have fatty acid in common but there are generally speaking a few different types of fats. Firstly, you have animal fats and plant fats.

The most common animal fats are lard and beef tallow but goose fat and chicken fat are also common. Many people feel uncomfortable using these fats for cleaning their bodies but luckily these fats make fantastic laundry soap.

With plants you can have seed oils, nut oils, or kernel oils, and vegetable oils (either from pressed fruit and vegetables or from the kernels of the fruit). Common ones include olive oil, almond oil, rapeseed oil, avocado oil, and argon oil.

These fats and oils all have their own properties and you typically combine a few different oils and fats to make soap. It's less common to use, for example, just coconut oil to make soap – it is a very fluffy soap that can be too cleansing for some people. Coconut oil will nearly always be balanced with an olive oil or a rapeseed oil to make it less greasy and easier on the skin.

When choosing a fat, you want to make a good balance of the characteristics you want form the finished product. These are cleansing, hardness, conditioning, and lather type.

Cleansing

The cleansing value of a fat tells you how much oil and dirt it will pick up and take off your body (or other things to be cleaned) when you use it. If the fat is too cleansing it will start to irritate the skin by taking away too much oil – some of which your body needs.

Unless you're making soap that is there to kill bacteria you can usually get away with soap that has a lower cleansing property.

Hardness

Hardness refers simply to how hard or soft soap will be – the end result might not vary hugely in how soft or hard they are but the big difference comes in the creation process. Hard fats harden quicker and are more difficult to put into swirls than soft soaps.

Conditioning

Conditioning soap allows skin and hair to retain moisture later on. This is a good property if you have skin that is easily dried out.

Lather type

You tend to have either bubbly lather or creamy lather and some fats don't produce much lather at all (especially if you don't add extra fat in). The two types of lather are largely to do with your preferences.

The type of fatty acid

One last technical thing to consider when choosing a fat is the types of fatty acid that are in it. Not all fatty acids are equal and some have quite different properties.

Early on you might not want to worry about these elements too much but when you decide to experiment finding out the fatty acid makeup of a fat will let you know what you should mix together to make a perfect soap.

Myristic acid

Myristic acid makes hard soap with high cleansing values and a bubbly lather. Too much myristic acid can make a drying soap.

Stearic acid

Stearic acid makes a hard soap with a strong creamy lather.

Oleic acid

Excellent for conditioning quality but reduces lather in a soap

Ricinolec acid

Ricinolec acid makes a mixed lather and has a good conditioning value.

Lauric acid

Lauric acid creates a hard bar with high cleaning values and a very bubbly lather.

Palmitic acid

Palmitic acid makes a hard soap with a creamy lather.

Linolenic acid

Good conditioning value.

Iodine value

The iodine value of a soap tells you how much iodine will end up in the soap using a specific fat. The more iodine you have a in soap the more conditioning a soap will be and the softer it will be.

Choosing a fat

So how does all this information work in practice? When you look at an oil or fat you can look up its chemical makeup to tell you what it will be good for.

If you take olive oil as an example it is 50 to 80% oleic acid, 3 to 20% linoleic acid, 7 to 20% palmitic acid, and 0 to 5% stearic acid. This means it makes a soap that is great for moisturizing and has a creamy to weak lather.

Coconut oil is 50% lauric acid and 20% myristic acid which will mean that it is an excellent hard and cleaning soap but it could be drying. Looking up the composition of different oils is fairly simple online and can tell you a lot about the kind of fat you want to use.

To give you a general picture we'll look at some of the most common fats here.

Tallow and lard

Tallow and lard are generally quite good all round soaps that don't need too much added to them. They tend to give a creamy lather and have good cleansing properties, but they also tend to produce a milky color and can benefit from being balanced out with a good conditioning fat.

Shea butter and cocoa butter

As the butter names implies these make a wonderfully creamy soap that is great for making lather. They are not fantastic at cleaning or necessarily at conditioning the skin but they make hard and long lasting soap.

Olive oil, rapeseed oil, castor oil, avocado oil, sunflower oil, hemp seed oil, almond oil, and safflower oil

These oils vary individually in their lather and cleansing abilities but they all have a fairly low lather and a low cleansing property meaning they are good to balance out drying soaps. They also typically have good conditioning properties.

Coconut oil, babassu oil, and palm kernel oil

These are the high cleansing values oils that often make for lots of bubbles in soap. Too much of these and they have a tendency to dry out skin.

Jojoba oil, meadowfoam oil, and beeswax

These oils can be used to heavily reduce lather in soap and is very waxy. It's good for making hard soap with a long shelf life but you'd typically only make them a small part of the fats you use.

Wheatgerm oil, emu oil, and rice bran oil

These are fairly mild oils and the main reason they are added to soaps is because they contain large amounts of vitamins in them. It's doubtful how much rubbing this on your skin does anything but it is worth considering.

The price of fat

You can probably tell from the list above that several types of oils and fats do similar things. If you're making soap for other people they're not likely to be too concerned whether you used olive oil or canola oil and they can have a similar finished product.

Castor, sunflower, and rapeseed oil are often cheaper than olive oil, palm oil is cheaper than coconut, and cocoa butter is cheaper than shea butter. If you are buying in bulk (as you should if you plan to make lots of soap) then a dollar saved per ounce can be quite significant.

When it comes to buying these things at a local store the effect can be even more dramatic as people often pay more for oils they perceive as luxurious. Coconut oil is an excellent example of this as it's often sold as an artisan product in smaller jars for an enormous markup.

With animal fat you'll often see big markups if you buy small amounts in places where it isn't popular. Lard for example is a very cheap product to make and in places where it is used widely in cooking (Europe, Mexico and the Southern USA) it can be bought for pennies. In some parts of the USA this almost worthless byproduct of a pig is sold as a luxury item.

Make sure to shop around and check for ethnic food suppliers for certain products at large discounts. For example, Asian food stores will often sell coconut oil for a fraction of the cost it is sold at regular supermarkets.

Discount and dollar stores are also good places to pick up cheap cooking oil.

Chapter 11: Best Homemade Soap Recipes

21. Heaven on Earth

*Cold process

Now, if you think that Mocha soap recipe is one-of-a-kind, well, you must try this one! Here we have Hot Chocolate Soap, for those who are ready to get to the next level of pleasure. Wonderful brown color, chocolate scent, and oils create a moisturizing mixture that your skin will fall in love with (and so will you!).

You need 40% olive oil, 20% lard or tallow, 25% coconut oil, and 5% castor oil. Per 1.1lbs (500 g) oils you need 2 tsp whole milk powder, 1 tbsp cocoa powder, 2 Tsp instant coffee granules, 2 tsp rhassoul clay, 5 g cocoa absolute, 2 tsp French red clay, and 10 g vanilla essential oil. Follow the steps for cold process. Once the mixture is like a pudding, add essential oils, clays, and powders.

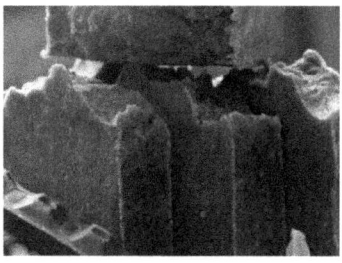

22. Honey and Dandelion Soap

*Cold process

Being one of the most popular soap recipes, it is clear that this soap has numerous benefits. Honey is antibacterial, and full of antioxidants, giving that wonderful summer glow to your skin. On the other hand, Dandelion treats acne and skin diseases, thus it is ideal for the problematic skin. Add to all that, benefits of other oils in this recipe and you get a top notch combination for your skin.

You need 14 ounces olive oil, 3 ounces sunflower oil, 8 ounces coconut oil, 2 ounces Shea butter, 1.5 ounces jojoba oil, 10 ounces dandelion tea, 1.5 ounces Tamanu oil, 4.07 ounces lye. When the mixture is consistent (trace) add a ½ ounce, raw honey.

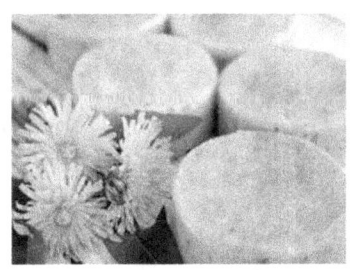

23. Beauty of France

*Melt and Pour method

Savon de Marseille gives rich and lavish showering experience, due to its remarkable scent and soothing properties. If you are a fan of lavender, like I am, then you will be thrilled with this mind-blowing combination. Whether you want to soothe yourself into sleep or boost your energy level the first thing in the morning, this soap can do both.

You need 5 lbs of olive oil soap base, 10 drops lavender essential oil, and 14 teaspoons of French clay.

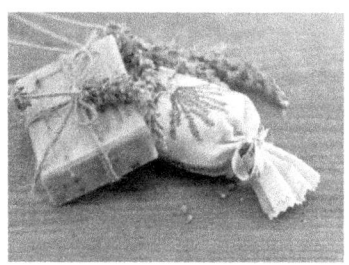

24. Sweet home

*Melt and Pour method

If you love classic, then you will also love this Honey Bee Soap. Honey will make your skin smooth and glow, while that well-known honey scent will remind you of your childhood. This soap also makes a great gift for Mother's Day, in case you want to surprise your mother. Trust me, her eyes will glisten with joy and nostalgia as soon as she breathes in this sweet smell.

You need 1 lb. block Honey Melt Base, 5 drops Baby Bee Buttermilk Fragrance Oil, 3 drops Vanilla White Color Stabilizer, 3 drops of Stained Glass Citrus Orange Colorant, and Honey Comb Bee Molds.

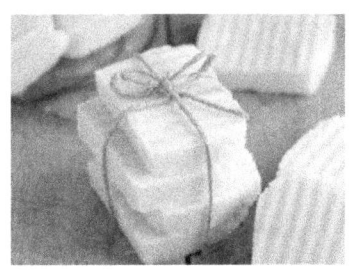

25. Simple yet Powerful

*Melt and pour process

Lemon Verbena and Lavender creates a strong combination, leaving your body relaxed and energized at the same time.

You need Goat's milk soap base, 10 drops of Lemon verbena, 10 drops Lavender essential oil, and dried lavender. If you want to give this soap to someone you love, buy a one-of-a-kind molds and voila – your present will look wonderful.

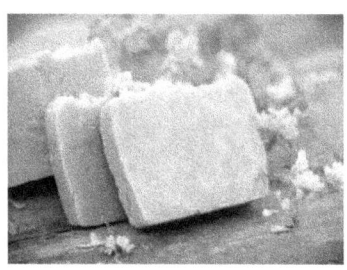

26. Bring the garden scents to your day

*Cold process

What better way to enjoy spring than breathing in strong garden scents while showering or taking a bath? Here we have a real deal for your body and mind, thanks to these ingredients. Let's see what ingredients make this soap so special. You need 4 ounces Avocado Oil, 28 ounces Olive Oil, 24 ounces Coconut Oil, 4 ounces Castor Oil, 2 ounces Mango Butter, 9.0 ounces lye and 19 ounces cooled mint tea.

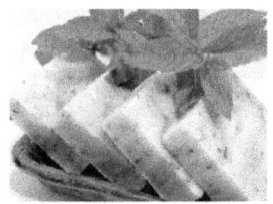

27. Who doesn't love that silky feel on their skin?

*Cold process

For those who long for a silk and rich shower time, this is the way to go. With

Shea butter, olive, coconut and castor oil, this soap turns an ordinary shower time into extraordinary experience. You will enjoy the luxury each time you use this soap.

You need 225 g Coconut Oil, 225 g Coconut oil, 90 g Castor oil, 360 g Olive oil, 342 g Distilled water, 123.75 g lye and 18 g silk peptide. You can also add 1/2tsp yellow soap colorant and essential oils of your choice.

Water as % of Oils = 38%

Super Fat/Discount = 5%

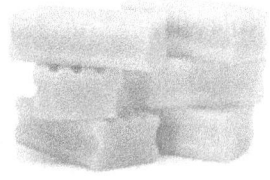

28. Old and New

Here we have another recipe for turning leftover soap bars into a fun and simple project. What's more, this project is economical, since you won't have to throw away the soap scraps like you normally would. Collect all the soap scraps and arrange them by colors and patterns. Don't be afraid to show how creative you can get.

Use a cheese grater for shredding soaps bars. You need to place them into large and separate bowls, to create colorful soap balls. You can add essential oils so that you can make balls of soap shreds much easier. When the soap shreds are divided into bowls, grab a handful of them and squeeze and roll them into a ball. Just make sure to press the shreds hard in order for a soap ball to harden. Next, add one more layer and repeat the process. You can repeat the process as long as you want until you get the desired soap size. If soap balls are made of fresh soap bars, then let them cure for a month.

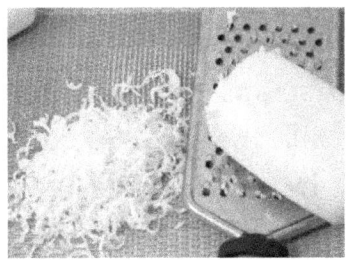

29. Jasmine

*Cold process

Here we have a romantic and moisturizing soap that will make your shower time lovely. You will be spoiled by that wonderful soap texture and smooth feel on your skin.

You need 40% olive oil, 10% shea butter, 25% coconut oil, 20% lard, and 5% castor oil. Per 500g oils: 1 tbsp kaolin clay, 0.32oz jasmine essential oil, 0.32oz ylang-ylang essential oil, 0.32oz rosewood wood essential oil, and 2 tsp titanium dioxide.

Lye at 5% discount

Follow the cold process soap making procedure and add clay and the titanium dioxide at trace.

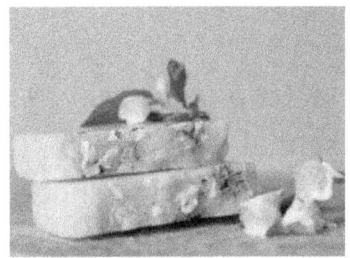

30. Honey and Carrot Soap

*Cold process

This Honey and Carrot soap is ideal for a mature skin, as it will make it silky and staple. This soap is a good choice for cleaning your face, but can also be used for your body. The reason why it is used for the face is that of beta carotene that will protect the skin from harmful sun's rays. Honey will bring shine to your skin and will help slow down the aging process.

You need 24 ounces coconut oil, 36 ounces olive oil, 2 ounces mango butter, 12 ounces palm kernel oil, 12.10 ounces of lye, 10 ounces palm fruit oil, 10 ounces freshly pressed carrot juice and an adequate amount of water to equal a total of 26 oz. of liquid.

At trace, stir in ½ Tbsp raw honey, 9 drops carrot seed essential oil, 1 Tbsp rosehip seed oil, 1Tbsp mango butter and ½ Tbsp Tamanu oil.

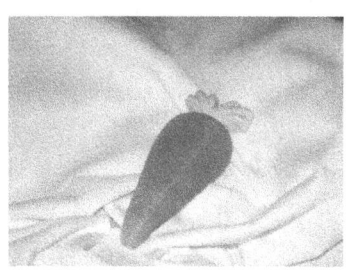

Chapter 12: Saponification Guide

In Plain English - How to Mix the Lye and Fats to Make Your Soap

This is the name of the chemical reaction that occurs when a fat is blended with an alkali substance - the end result is that soap is created.

Getting Your Lye On

We have already discussed a little about the fats that you will use so let's talk a little about lye now. Lye is alkaline in nature and its scientific name is Sodium Hydroxide. It may also be called Caustic Soda and you will get it at a hardware store. Do be careful to only buy 100% pure Caustic Soda/ Lye/ Sodium Hydroxide.

Now, just to give you an idea of how dangerous lye can be, a lye water bath can be used to clean flesh off bones. There was, indeed a famous murdered in the 1800's who laid his victim's body in a lye bath in order to dissolve them. He was finally caught because their teeth did not dissolve as well.

I am not saying that to put you off, the strength that we use in soap is a lot weaker than would be used for the above processes but I do need you to understand that lye is not to be trifled with at all.

The fumes are toxic and can cause damage to the inner flesh of the mouth, nose and respiratory tract if it is ingested. If the lye water falls onto the skin, it causes serious burns and, if ingested, can kill. Even the crystals themselves should be handled with care - the minute they are mixed with water, even if that means sweat on the skin, they can cause burns.

Lye can take the form of pellets, flakes, power or beads and you can choose whichever of these you prefer - as long as it is 100% lye, it does not matter because we will be dissolving them anyway. I personally prefer using flakes and I buy only small amounts at a time to avoid the need to store dangerous chemicals at home.

So, if lye is so dangerous, why on earth to we put it in soap? The chemical reaction of the oils and lye causes them to change nature completely. The lye is largely neutralized in the process and, at the end of it, we have a great cleaning agent.

Note that I said that the lye is largely neutralized. The raw soap needs to be left to cure for at least four to six weeks in order to render the lye completely neutral. This process can be sped up by using a hot-process soap making recipe but that is not something that we will deal with in this book. Personally I find that the curing period goes by pretty fast and I prefer to see how the batch ages. Imagine selling a batch of freshly made soap and having it come back because it is moldy. If the soap is left to cure, you have plenty of time to see whether mold will develop or not.

Soap making is something that is both difficult to get wrong and easy to get wrong - it all depends on how well you have adhered to the proper ratios and whether or not you have followed the correct processes. As long as you always have the right proportion of oil to lye, you will not be able to go too far wrong. The process of converting an oil into soap using lye is referred to as saponification. In order to determine how much lye you will need, you will need to know the saponification value of the oils that you intend to use, unless you are following someone else's recipe. You can look up all the different saponification values (SAP) on the internet and the calculation is fairly simple from there. Alternatively, you can find a number of online calculators that will do all the work for you.

How Much Lye Should I Be Using?

Let's say that you've chosen to use a base of olive oil. It has an SAP of 0.134. You then need to multiply the weight of the oil that you are intending to use by the SAP in order to work out how much lye you are going to actually need. Let's say you've decided to use 5 ounces of olive oil, for example, the calculation will be:

5 x 0.134 = 0.67. You will thus need around 0.67 ounces of lye to convert the oil to soap. If you want a more moisturizing soap, you can reduce the lye content by about 5% so that some of the oil is not saponified. This is known as super-fatting and makes the end result more moisturizing. The bar will not be as long-lasting though and more prone to going rancid. I do not advise messing with these numbers too much initially though – especially while you are learning.

Chapter 13: Time For Some Homemade Recipes!

Of course, this book will not completely serve its purpose without any sample of recipes that you can use and get new ideas.

Now, let's start!

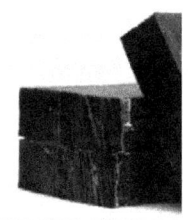

1.)Tea Tree and Activated Charcoal Soap –

It is most effective for individuals that have oily skin. This soap is has sleek and quite sexy because of its alluring color. It has healing properties of tea tree oil with the detoxifying properties of activated charcoal.

The ingredients are:

☐ 12 Bar Rectangle Silicone Mold

☐ 1.8 ounce of Castor Oil (5%)

☐ 9 ounce of Coconut Oil (25%)

☐ 14.4 ounce of Olive Oil (40%)

☐ 9 ounce of Palm Oil (25%)

☐ 1.8 ounce of Tamanu Oil (5%)

☐ 5.1 ounce of Sodium Hydroxide Lye

☐ 10.1 ounce of Distilled Water (15% water discount)

☐ 1.7 ounce of Tea Tree Essential Oil

☐ 2 Tablespoon of Activated Charcoal

☐ Optional: 2 tablespoon of Sodium Lactate

How to do it:

1.)Gradually add the lye to the water and delicately mix. Stop when the mixture is clear. That would mean that the lye is dissolved. Place it still in a safe spot.

2.)Completely melt the olive oil, coconut oil, and the palm oil, and the Tamanu oil (keep in mind that you must completely melt the essential oils before mixing). After the lye-water mixture has completely cooled to around 130 degrees, you can now add the lye water to the oils and stick blend until the trace becomes thin. On the other hand, if you like a bar that is harder, then you might want to give it some sodium lactate on the cooled mixture. Just utilize 1 tsp. of sodium lactate per lbs. of essential oils for this recipe.

3.)Now, add two tablespoon of activated charcoal to the mixture. Don't forget to use the stick blender to constantly tap down the activated charcoal to start to mix it into the batter. If you just turn on the stick mixer suddenly, the activated charcoal could poof into the air. Just gradually pulse the stick blender to integrate the activated charcoal.

4.)Then incorporate the tea tree oil to the soap, and use your stick blender to mix and stir the oil fully.

5.)Continue on stirring the mixture for a few more seconds in order to ensure that the ingredients are fully mixed. When the soap is in a medium trace, and is still pourable, go ahead and pour the batter into the individual cavities of the twelve bar rectangle mold.

6.)Squirt the top of the soap using a 99% isopropyl alcohol to preclude soda ash. Put on a heater, and insulate the soap for around 30 minutes. Then turn off the heater, and leave the soap insulated for about 24 hours.

7.)Make the soap to stay in the mold for another three to four days since this soap has plenty of essential oils which might need up to a week in the mold. Don't hasten it because once the soap is hard enough, you can now unmold and cure it for about 4 weeks. Have fun!

Pure Coconut Oil Soap –

this kind of soap is good for cleansing and moisturizing your skin. By utilizing the excellent process of superfatting, extra coconut oil is incorporated than the lye, making a bar that has extra fattiness and thus increases moisturizing properties.

Ingredients:

☐ 5 ounce of coconut oil

- [ ] 5 ounce of lye
- [ ] 13 ounce of distilled water
- [ ] 1 ounce of essential oils

Tools:

- [ ] Protective goggles and gloves
- [ ] Silicone Mold
- [ ] Parchment Paper
- [ ] Spoon blender
- [ ] Crock pot
- [ ] Thermometer
- [ ] Digital Scale
- [ ] Measuring Cups
- [ ] Small bowls
- [ ] Disposable spoon (w/ a long handle)
- [ ] Rubber Spatula

Here's how to do it:

1.)Start by scaling your ingredients and setting up your crockpot into low

2.)Add water to a medium-sized cup and bring it outside along with your lye and spoon mixer, of course you must be wearing a goggles and a pair of gloves. Remember that inhaling the lye mixture's vapor is harmful. Also, keep in mind that you're pouring lye into the water, and not the other way around. As discussed earlier, the mixing of lye and water will get very hot. Wait until the mixture is clear then proceed to the next step.

3.)Put the coconut oil in a container, preferably a pan and heat it up to 130F. Ensure that your thermometer will not be touching the bottom part of the pan when you are reading the temperature.

4.)Now put the coconut oil to the crockpot and set it to low.

5.) Add the lye to the crockpot and stir for a couple of times.

6.) Now mix the mixture using stick blender and get it into trace. This happens when the mixture becomes similar to a light pudding.

Let the mixture cook on low and cover it. Monitor it consistently. If it rises up the sides and looks like it might ooze, just stir it and the volume will get lessen.

7.) If the soap seems like a semi translucent vaseline that has no oil puddles in the middle, it's now ready.

8.) If you are planning on adding essential oils, wait until the soap cools a bit then start adding whatever you desire.

9.) Transfer the mixture by scooping it into the mold and let it cool. Put it in fridge if you want to harden it fast.

10.) Coconut oil bars are difficult to cut if you dry it for too long, that's why it's always better if you cut it as soon as it's firm. It's ideal if you cure them for around 2-3 week to develop its soap properties completely.

2.) Aloe Vera Soap

– aloe vera can soothe burns, treat acnes, has anti-aging properties, a great moisturizer, and can even help heal wounds! Most likely, it is one of the most beneficial and ideal ingredient for making a soap. What you want do is simple. If you have an aloe vera plant, just get the gel from it, or if you don't have any plant, you can buy some organic aloe vera gel, and mix it with coconut oil, olive oil, lard, shea butter, and of course lye.

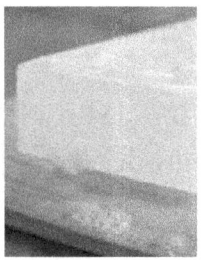

The ingredients are:

- ☐ 7.5 ounce of mineral water
- ☐ 3 ounce of lye
- ☐ 1.5 pounds of olive oil
- ☐ 0.4 oz beeswax
- ☐ 1.8 oz aloe vera juice
- ☐ 0.18 oz mint essential oil

Here are the steps:

1.)Pour the H20 to a desired-sized pan, and gradually add lye, stir it gently until the mixture becomes clear. As usual, make sure you are wearing a pair of gloves, and goggles. Make sure the caustic soda substance is around 130F.

2.)In different pan, start heating olive oil up to 130F, gradually adding beeswax while stirring the olive oil and beeswax mixture slowly.

3.)Get the olive oil and beeswax mixture from heat, and start adding the lye mixture and stir gently.

4.)Stir consistently after every 10 minutes until it gets a consistency just like of that light pudding.

5.)Now, start stirring the aloe vera juice and your chosen essential oils for approximately one minute.

6.)You can now start pouring the mixture into a mold. Make sure you tap the mold in order to eliminate air bubbles.

7.)Cover the mold with the mixture and let it cool for around two days. Get the cover, and let it sit still for one extra day.

8.) Get the hardened soap from the mold and wait for the next day. After that, you can cut it as you desire.

9.)For best results, cure the finished product for about one month to ensure its soap properties to appear.

3.)Coffee Soap –

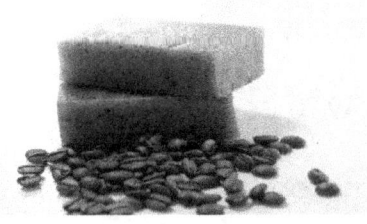

In various ways, this soap seems very interesting. Coffee soap has excellent aroma. First and foremost, you must know that this recipe is a melt and pour recipe that's why we will be a goat's milk soap as a base, and an almond oil for conditioning, your chosen fragrance, and of course some coffee grounds, I'm sure you'll get extra fresh and vibrant throughout the day!

Ingredients:

☐ 1.5 lbs Organic Goat's Milk Soap

☐ 1 Tablespoon of fresh ground coffees

☐ 1 Teaspoon of Almond Oil

☐ 1 – 1.5 Teaspoons of Fragrance such as cinnamon, and vanilla

Here's how to do it:

1.) Cut the organic goat's milk soap into pieces

2.) Delicately melt the chunks on a low to medium heat

3.) After melting, quickly remove from heat and mix in your coffee grounds, chosen fragrance, and almond oil

4.) Then pour into the mold

5.) Spray some rubbing alcohol in order to prevent air bubbles.

6.) After ridding of air bubbles, you can now begin the hardening process. Place in the fridge if you want to speed up the process.

7.) If you put the product into the fridge, wait up until 1-2 days. For normal cooling process in a cool dry place, wait up until 4-7 days for complete hardening process.

8.) Obviously, if they are fully hardened, you can now pop them out from the molds and store in an air-tight containers. For this recipe, there's no need for curing, and you can already use if desired.

5.)Honey Oatmeal Soap –

One of the soap that I've made that has deep rich aroma which makes me want to wash my hands again and again.

Ingredients:

☐ 2 tbsp. of honey

☐ 2 tbsp. and 1 tsp. quick oats

☐ ½ lbs. of goat's milk soap

☐ soap colorants

☐ measuring cup

☐ knife

☐ silicone molds

☐ spoon for mixing

How To Do It:

☐ Get a coffee grinder to grind up 2 tbsp. of oatmeal. Make sure it becomes a fine powder.

☐ Cut the goat's milk soap into cubes, and put it into the measuring cup.

☐ Melt the soap base in a microwave for around 30 seconds, and stir after microwaving. It is ideal to completely melt it for a total of 1 minute, with 30 seconds interval. Make sure not to over-heat the soap base because it could deteriorate the soap base's properties.

☐ Get it out from your microwave and you can now add whatever ingredients you desired, of course you should not forget the honey and ground oatmel.

☐ Make sure you stir it nice. If you ever purchased any soap colorant, you should give it two drops of red and 6 drops of yellow in order to get a pale yellow color.

☐ Meantime, sprinkle tsp. of oatmeal flakes on the molds. Then pour the soap liquid mixture according to the size of the mold.

☐ Make sure you avoid moving the soap mold just after pouring the liquid soap because it could affect the appearance of the soap. Place a tray beforehand just in case.

☐ Don't move the mold with the poured liquid soap for up to 20 minutes. After that, you can now freely place it in a cool dry place to hardened.

☐ Remove the soap from the silicone molds, and let it sit again for a couple of days (ideally 4 days) to fully dry and hardened.

☐ After the complete hardening, wrap it with your chosen style of wrapping, and you can now freely give it or sell it to anyone as you wish.

6.)Lemon Green Tea Soap –

this DIY soap is excellent for maintaining vibrant skin. On the other hand, its Green Tea ingredient is has tons of antioxidants which can aid lessen skin deterioration and preclude premature aging of your skin. Meanwhile its Lemon ingredient is loaded of benefits just like green tea. The ascorbic acid it possess aids to fight skin aging. Vitamin C also minimizes acnes. This soap has also glycerin which is good for moisturizing your skin

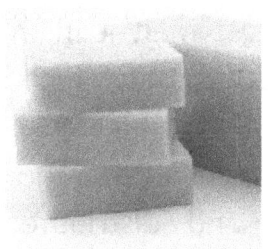

The ingredients:

☐ 1 lbs. of melt & pour glycerin soap

☐ 2 tablespoon of green tea poweder

☐ 3/4 tablespoon of essential lemon oil

☐ Molds (preferably silicone for easy removal)

How To Do It:

☐ Cut the soap base into little cubes, put the chopped cubes into a bowl that will not melt in a microwave (batter bowl is good), and place the bowl with the chopped soap inside the microwave.

☐ Now, don't over-cooked your soap base because it could damage its soap properties. Just melt it in the microwave for around 30 seconds, high temp for 2-3 intervals of 30 seconds. Make sure you stir the soap base for each interval to remove air bubbles and distribute it properly. Observe if its fully melted by checking if there are still any soap base chunks.

☐ Just after removing the batter bowl from your microwave, immediately put in your green tea powder as well as the essential lemon oil. Mix it thoroughly but make sure you are not mixing it when its entering its hardening stage.

☐ Carefully pour the liquefied soap base mixture into your silicone mold. Make sure you cool it down for a few hours. Then remove it from the mold, and lastly cure it for around 3-4 days.

☐ In order not to lose its aroma, you must make sure that you store it in an airtight container until you decide to use it.

COCONUT MILK SHAMPOO BARS-
With its high lauric acid content, coconut milk ensures this shampoo bar recipe has a bubbly lather and extra creamy feel, while jojoba oil adds a touch of luxury that's fantastic for promoting healthy, shiny hair.

Ingredients:

- [ ] 4.5 ounce of mineral water
- [ ] 3.85 ounce of lye
- [ ] 4 ounce of full-fat coconut oil
- [ ] 7.5 ounce of virgin coconut oil
- [ ] 12 ounce of olive oil
- [ ] 3.5 ounce of almond oil
- [ ] 4 ounce of castor oil
- [ ] 1 ounce of jojoba oil

How To Do It:

- [ ] First and foremost you must be wearing your goggles and gloves. Delicately mix the lye into the mineral water. After that, make sure you set aside the lye-water mixture for around 35 minutes or just until its temperature drops for around 100°F.

- [ ] While waiting, start melting your full-fat coconut oil, and carefully add the other essential oils. Start adding the coconut milk in order to warm the oils. Try using an immersion mixer for a couple of seconds until fully mixed.

☐ Start adding your cooled lye-water solution into your warm oils, and the coconut milk mixture. Stir the mixture until it attains a light consistency.

☐ After getting the right consistency without any left-over chunks, you can now pour the liquid into a silicon mold. Ideally, you might want to cover it with a freezer paper. Make sure you monitor the hardening phase of the soap, and spot it if it's starting to get some cracks. If it starts breaking, uncover the mold, and transfer it into a cooler place.

☐ Wait for up to 2 days, then remove it from its mold. After removing, wait for another day in order to harden completely. Then chop it as you desire.

7.) Dandelions Soap Bar –

this product is great for newbie soap crafter. Dandelions have various medicinal properties like aiding to relieve stomach aching, and helping you to remove surplus water from your body. If not for soap making, this dandelions would be great for making pestos and salads!

Ingredients:

☐ 6.08 oz. of coconut oil

☐ 6.40 oz. of dandelion fused with essential olive oil

☐ 3.20 oz. of shea butter

☐ 0.32 oz. of castor oil

☐ 2 tbsp. of natural honey

☐ 6.08 oz. of mineral water

☐ 2.31 oz. of lye.

Tools:

- Protective Goggles and gloves
- Large plastic bowl
- Spoon (preferably wooden)
- Stick blender
- Crockpot
- Safe bowl oven
- Kitchen scale
- Digital Thermometer
- Silicone molds

How To Do It:

1.)Start by measuring your essential oils with their weight, then put them in your crockpot. Meanwhile delicately melt your coconut oil and shea butter all together, the mixed in with your essential oils in the crockpot.

2.) Mix the ingredients in the crockpot delicately. Ideally, you would want your oils to cool down for around 80 degrees F. Make use of your digital thermometer to monitor the temperature. Keep in mind that if the essentials became too hot, they may not attain the right consistency.

3.) Now you can now add your lye to the water. Make sure that you are careful doing this task since you are dealing with a potential harmful chemical. Before adding the lye-water mixture to the other ingredients, make sure that you cool it down for at least 25 minutes.

4.) After cooling down your lye-water mixture, add it to your essential oils and gently stir to mix them. By means of a stick blender, mix the mixture until it attains a pudding like texture. This is now what you call a trace. After achieving the trace, cover the crockpot and turn it on low, and cook the mixture for about 1 hour.

5.) After 1 hour of cooking, mix them to fuse all the glycerin that formed on the upper portion of the ingredients. After cleaning the cooked mixture, you can now turn off the crock pot, and ready your silicone molds.

6.) And lastly, add your natural honey, and gently stir it with the cooked mixture. After delicately mixing, you can now pour it carefully into the molds. Cool it for about 2 days, then remove. Cool it for additional 1 day for complete hardening. Chopped it accordingly. Make sure you store it in an open area so that the air can help it with its curing process.

8.) Honey and Milk Soap –

this product is mostly likely my favorite. It just smells good, and apparently it has tons of skin benefits particularly because of the honey ingredient mixed within it. Honey is good for clarifying, moisturizing, and soothing your skin. It also has excellent antibacterial property that's why it's good for threatening aging, and acnes. This DIY homemade soap will take quite some time for the hardening process, but the actual project will only take you for more or less 10 minutes.

Here's What You Need:

- Soap Base (Ideally goat's milk)

- Silicone Mold (You can try for a honeycomb shape)

- Natural Honey

- Measuring Cup

- Soap Colorant (Red or Yellow is good)

How To Do It:

1.) Use around 1 pound of the goat's milk soap base, or as you desired if you are planning to make a large bloc of honey and milk soap. The soap base is soft so you can chop it easily by simply using a kitchen knife. Chop the soap base, and place it into a measuring cup, and start melting the base in your microwave. Keep in mind that you should get it out from the microwave every 30 seconds, and stir it again to make sure that it melts fully, then put it back. Do this for at least 3 rounds.

2.)After melting the soap base fully, put in some 3 tbsp. of natural honey, and a tinge of yellow soap coloring. You can also add whatever color you are thinking of to give the final product a vibrant color.

3.)Now you can start pouring the mixed liquefy into your honeycomb mold. Sit it still until it cools down. Since we only used a small mold, the cooling process will only take for around 2 hours depending on the temperature of the room the soap was placed.

4.)Carefully remove the soap from its mold, and let it sit for additional day for the curing process.

5.)Wrap it, or use it as you wish.

9.)Creamy Avocado Soap Bar –

I've found some argan oil, about 6 oz. and have decided to make use of it. I tried utilizing it with avocado oil, and guess what? The product is heavenly nice!

Here's What You Need:

- 8 oz. of Avocado Essential Oil
- 8 oz. of Babassu Essential Oil
- 7 oz. of Olive Essential Oil
- 6 oz. of Coconut Essential Oil
- 6 oz. of Argan Essential Oil
- 3 oz. of Castor Essential Oil
- 5.3. oz. of Lye
- 6.75 oz. of Mineral Water
- 5 oz. of Pureed Avocado
- 15g. of Lime Oil

- 12g. of Grapefruit Oil
- 10g. of lavender oil
- 5g. of sweet basil oil
- 6g. of Litsea Cubeba oil
- ½ tsp. of green and yellow oxide colorant

How To Do It:

1.)Grate out a piece of avocado. Weight the grated fruit out of four oz. and then smoothen it by means of a stick blender.

2.)On the other hand measure your essential oils, and get your lye solution ready.

3.)Get your ½ tsp. of your yellow and green oxide into your measuring cup. Mix it with about tablespoon of your essential oils.

4.)Now, add your smoothen avocado into your mixing pot and blend it along with the other ingredients. At the same time, carefully add your lye solution into your essential oils. Mix until it reached trace. After attaining trace, pour a third of your ingredients into your measuring cup alongside with your colorant. You can also add whatever fragrance you have at hand during this process.

5.)Now, intricately mix all of your ingredients. Pour a small amount of your green colored soap to your main batch on each corners, and a bit in the center. You don't need any additional mixing in your pot since it will automatically make an excellent swirl after pouring the soap.

6.)After that, fill the next layer with the surplus green soap mixture. Don't worry if the process breaks the lower part of the soap.

7.)Now, start pouring the rest of the mixture into the mold. If your soap is hardening, you must pour higher.

8.) And lastly, hardened the avocado with argan oil soap for about 2 days. After removing it from mold, it is better if you leave it for another 2 days to completely harden it.

9.) Chopped it accordingly and cure it. Wrap it or use it as you desire.

10.) Lavender Lotion Bar –

this soap is excellent for moisturizing and conditioning your skin especially if its always dry. In addition, it is good for relaxing and soothing aromatherapy convenience. It's also good for disinfecting your skin, and heals burns.

What You Need:

☐ ½ cup of shea butter

☐ 1 cup of coconut oil

☐ 1 cup of beeswax

☐ 16 drops of lavender essential oil

Silicone molds (Ideally a flower or oval mold)

How To Do It:

1.)Melt your cup of beeswax in a small pan along with your coconut oil until it gets the right liquid consistency.

2.)Now, mix in the shea butter until it is fully dissolved.

3.)After all the premixing, you can now remove from heat your melted beeswax and coconut oil and start adding your essential oils. You must start with just 5 drops, and gradually add drops until you get the right fragrance based on your preference. Make sure you are not putting so much drops into it, otherwise you might not be able to use it because of the strong smell.

4.)After achieving the right fragrance with your lavender essential oils, you can now pour the mixture into your silicone mold and cool it for about 4 days.

5.)After 4 days of hardening, remove it from the mold, and place in a cool dry location. Don't try storing your finished product in a room temperature since it could melt.

11.) Orange Clove Soap Bar –

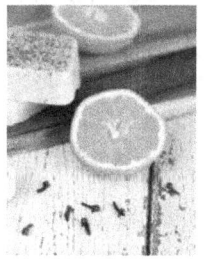

if you didn't know, there are loads of sin benefits from orange clove soap. Clove and orange essential oils are loaded of antiseptic properties and are excellent for ridding of acne problems. If not for soap making, orange is actually good for improving your mood, while clove is good for treating anxiety. You mustn't also forget that orange is great since it has good anti-aging properties.

What You Need:

- 1 lbs. of goat's milk soap base
- 2 teaspoon of ground cloves
- 2 teaspoon of dried orange skin
- 30 drops of orange oil
- 15 drops of clove oil
- Silicone mold

How To Do It:

1.) Chop the goat's milk soap base and place the chopped soap base in a batter bowl. Before putting in the microwave, add the dried chopped orange peel, and the ground cloves.

2.)Place in the microwave for 50 seconds on high, then stir it, then remove for stirring, and place it again for another 50 seconds the soap base completely melts.

3.)Remove from the microwave and blend it until the ingredients on the mixture are all dispersed. Mix until you get the right liquid consistency just like a pudding.

4.)After achieving the trace, you can start adding your essential oils, and mix well. After all the mixing, start pouring the mixture into your silicone molds.

5.)Wait for 3-4 days in order to fully harden. After that, remove it from the mold, and cure it for additional 2 days. After the curing process, seal the finished product in an airtight container.

Vanilla and Brown Sugar Soap –

with the use of brown sugar in this product, it will give a gorgeous translucent color, with a sweet scent improved due to the vanilla essential oil.

What Do You Need:

☐ 1 pounds of glycerine soap base

☐ 2 teaspoon of vanilla essential oil

☐ 2 tablespoon of brown sugar

☐ Silicone molds

☐ Rubbing alcohol

How To Do It:

1.)First, chopped the glycerine soap base into pieces, and put them into a large batter bowl.

2.)Place it into the microwave for about 40 seconds. After the initial melting, remove it, and blend well, then place it again the microwave for another 40 seconds, and repeat blending it until it completely melts.

3.)Now you can now fuse your brown sugar, and vanilla essential oil in a separate container. After mixing the two ingredients, you can now add it into the melted soap base.

4.)After mixing the essential oils and soap base, you can now pour the mixture into your silicone molds.

5.)After pouring, it is better if you spray it with little amount of rubbing alcohol in order to get rid of any air bubbles which could affect the soap properties of the product.

6.)After spraying some alcohol, place your silicone mold with the mixture inside it in a cool dry place in order to cool down for about 2 hours. Then you can remove it from its mold and cure it for 3-4 days.

7.)Wrap in an airtight container, or use it if you desire.

12.) Banana and Yogurt Soap Bar –

this soap bar is made from pure banana which is rich in both vitamin A and potassium. This product is excellent for those individuals who have dry skin. On the other hand, the yogurt powder will serve to soothe your skin. Take note that this recipe has organic flax seed essential oil which has essential fatty acids, vitamin B, E, and some minerals. It is even good for those people who have sensitive skin.

What Do You Need:

- 1.6 ounce of coconut essential oil
- 1.6 ounce of castor essential oil
- 4.8 ounce of babassu essential oil
- 3.2. ounce of cocoa butter
- 17.6 ounce of olive oil
- 1.6 ounce of shea butter
- 1.7 ounce of flax seed essential oil
- 10 ounce of mineral water
- 5 ounce of Lye

- 1 ounce of sodium lactate
- 0.4 ounce of yogurt powder
- 0.5 ounce of banana powder
- 2 ounce of desired fragrance oil

How To Do It:

1.)First and foremost, you must be familiar now of the cold making process before doing this recipe. Of course, you must stick with all the basic safety precautions while working with caustic soda, a.k.a. lye.

2.)Now start by measuring the amount of water, and place it into a heat safe bowl because you will be mixing it with the lye afterwards. Now weigh out your caustic soda relative with the amount of water you measured.

3.)Carefully pour your lye into your water. Ideally, you want to do this process in a fine-ventilated area. Stir the mixture until you get a clear lye-water mixture, and set it aside for later use.

4.)After working with the lye mixture, start measuring your essential oils, and butters according to the ingredients recipe above. Heat these soapmaking oils until fully melted.

5.)Now, after your lye-water mixture, and your soapmaking oils got a temperature of around 95 degree F, it is now the time to start the main event!

6.)Measure your sodium lactate, and mix it into your lye mixture.

7.)After that, measure your banana and yogurt powders, and your fragrance oil (if you have). After weighing them, add them into the melted mixture, and fuse them all with the use of a stick blender.

8.)Now, get the lye-water mixture, and carefully pour it into your completely melted ingredients.

9.) Using a stick blender, mix all the ingredients along with the lye until you achieve trace. After that, you can now start pouring your banana and yogurt batter into your silicone mould's cavities.

10.) After pouring the mixture, it is better if you cover it with a parchment paper, and keep in a safe cool, dry place for 3-4 days.

11.) After hardening, remove the soap from the silicone molds, and wait for another 1-2 days to completely harden all the sides of the soap.

12.) After your soap fully hardened, cure it now for about 5 weeks. After curing, obliviously the soap is now ready for use, gifting, or selling.

Chapter 14: Recipes

Refer to details of the soap making process in the cold process section. However, here are the steps again for simplicity.

Weigh your ingredients using the scale

Add the lye to the pitcher containing water (not the other way around) and stir to make a lye solution

Heat the oils to 110 F

Add the lye solution to the oil when they are at 100 F and stir

Using a stick blender, mix the mixture in short bursts until you achieve trace

Add your fragrance or essential oils

Pour your soap mixture into your chosen mold and let it harden for 12-24 hours to solidify

You can use the soap immediately, but it is better to let it cure for 3-4 weeks

Don't forget to adequately wash the equipment and utensils used

Use this method for all the following recipes.

Prep time for all recipes is appx. 60-120 minutes.

Quick and simple 4-oil soap recipe

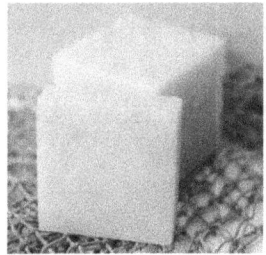

The oils

7.5 ounces olive oil

6.5 ounces palm oil

1.3 ounces castor oil

6.5 ounces coconut oil

The lye mixture

3.1 ounces lye

8 ounces water

Personal additions

1 ounce of your favorite fragrance oil or any essential oil blend

Petals or exfoliants if desired

Olive oil soap for sensitive baby skin

The high olive oil concentration makes this recipe soft and mild on your baby's skin. It is nourishing as well. However, the soap may need longer time to cure as the olive oil will make the soap take its time to harden but it will be worth it in the end as it will appeal to your baby's soft and sensitive skin.

This recipe can make 12 bars, 3.6 pounds each

The oils

2.1 ounces 5% castor oil

6.2 ounces 15% coconut oil

28.7 ounces regular or infused 70% olive oil

4.1 ounces 10% shea butter

For the lye solution

5.48 ounces Lye

10.6 ounces water

2 teaspoons of sugar added to the lye solution

1.5 teaspoons of salt added to the lye solution

Additions

Optional, depending on how sensitive your baby's skin is

1.8 ounces fragrance or essential oil

Creamy and luxurious soap recipe

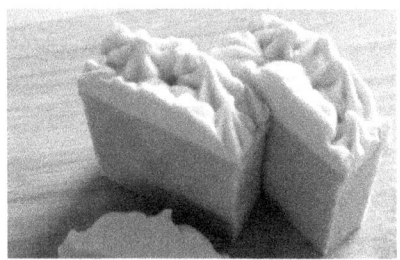

Any soap recipe that includes milk is known to be super moisturizing and gives your soap a luxurious creamy touch. You can replace the water in your lye solution with milk either entirely or use half water and half milk when dissolving the lye. You can also use powdered milk that you add during the trace step. Either ways, this is a wonderful recipe if you suffer from dry skin.

The oils

2.75 ounces 14% almond oil

1 ounce 5% castor oil

5.3 ounces 27% olive oil

5.3 ounces 27% palm oil

5.3 ounces 27% coconut oil

For the lye solution

2.8 ounces of lye

5.9 ounces of water

Additional

1 ounce fragrance oil

Note: You can make half the 5.9 water and half of it milk. If you decide to use liquid milk, add the milk with the lye solution. If you decided to use heavy cream instead of milk, add it with the oils.

Conclusion

I am extremely excited to pass this information along to you, and I am so happy that you now have read and can hopefully implement these strategies going forward.

I hope this book was able to help you understand soap making and how to start whipping up your own bars of organic soaps at home.

The next step is to get started using this information and to hopefully live a healthier and more fulfilling life!

Please don't be someone who just reads this information and doesn't apply it, the strategies in this book will only benefit you if you use them!

If you know of anyone else that could benefit from the information presented here please inform them of this book.

Thank you and good luck!

www.ingramcontent.com/pod-product-compliance
Lightning Source LLC
Chambersburg PA
CBHW071826080526
44589CB00012B/925